DATE DUE

DRUGS, ALCOHOL, PREGNANCY AND PARENTING

To Joel, Ari, and Gabriel

Children bring out the best in us all.

DRUGS, ALCOHOL, PREGNANCY AND PARENTING

Edited by

Ira J Chasnoff, MD

Associate Professor of Pediatrics and Psychiatry
and Behavioral Sciences
Northwestern University Medical School
Director, Perinatal Center for Chemical Dependence
Northwestern Memorial Hospital
Chicago, Illinois, USA

KLUWER ACADEMIC PUBLISHERS
DORDRECHT / BOSTON / LONDON

Distributors

for the United States and Canada: Kluwer Academic Publishers, PO Box 358, Accord Station, Hingham, MA 02018-0358, USA
for all other countries: Kluwer Academic Publishers Group, Distribution Center, PO Box 322, 3300 AH Dordrecht, The Netherlands

British Library Cataloguing in Publication Data

Drugs, alcohol, pregnancy and parenting.
    1. Man. Foetuses. Effects of alcohol
    consumption of mothers   2. Man.
    Foetuses. Effects of drug addiction
    of mothers
    I. Chasnoff, Ira J., *1947–*
    618.3'2

    ISBN 0-7462-0095-1

Contents

THE WHITE HOUSE

September 8, 1987

Dear Friends:

Although I cannot be with you, this
brings my warm greetings to all those
participating in the National Conference
on Drug Use in Pregnancy. I am
delighted to serve as Honorary Chairman
of this very important conference.

Substance abuse has become a national
epidemic in our country and no where is
its impact more profound than on the
lives of innocent children born to women
who abuse alcohol and drugs. Through
the tireless dedication of individuals
such as those gathered here today, an
intensive cooperative effort has been
launched to educate women about the
potentially fatal effects of drug use
to unborn children.

You have my heartfelt thanks for your
loving dedication to this new
generation of Americans. With best
wishes for continued success,

        Sincerely,

        Nancy Reagan

National Conference on Drug
  Use in Pregnancy

List of Contributors

William T Atkins
Director, Illinois Department of
Alcoholism and Substance Abuse
100 W. Randolph Street
Chicago, Illinois 60601, USA

Rita Allen Brennan
Supervisor, Special Care Nursery
St. Joseph Hospital and Health
Care Center
Chicago, Illinois 60614, USA

Kayreen A Burns
Assistant Professor of Psychiatry
and Behavioral Sciences and
Pediatrics
Northwestern University Medical
School
Child Development Clinic
Prentice Women's Hospital
333 East Superior Street
Chicago, Illinois 60611, USA

William J Burns
Assistant Professor of Psychiatry
and Behavioral Sciences and
Pediatrics
Child Development Clinic
Prentice Women's Hospital
333 East Superior Street
Chicago, Illinois 60611, USA

Ellen Gould Chadwick
Assistant Professor of Pediatrics
Division of Infectious Diseases
Children's Memorial Hospital
2300 Children's Plaza
Chicago, Illinois 60614, USA

Ira J Chasnoff
Associate Professor of Pediatrics
and Psychiatry and Behavioral
Sciences
Northwestern University Medical
School
Director, Perinatal Center for
Chemical Dependence
Northwestern Memorial Hospital
215 East Chicago Avenue
Chicago, Illinois 60611, USA

Amin N Daghestani
Associate Professor of Psychiatry
Loyola University Stritch School of
Medicine
2160 South First Avenue
Maywood, Illinois 60153, USA

Loretta P Finnegan
Professor of Pediatrics and
Psychiatry and Human Behavior
Jefferson Medical College
Thomas Jefferson University
Department of Pediatrics, Family
Center Program
Philadelphia, Pennsylvania 19107,
USA

Dan R Griffith
Perinatal Center for Chemical
Dependence
215 East Chicago Avenue
Chicago, Illinois 60611, USA

Sandy Hoffman
Outreach Education Coordinator,
Women and Infants Health
Prentice Women's Hospital
333 East Superior Street
Chicago, Illinois 60611, USA

Louis G Keith
Professor of Obstetrics and
Gynecology
Northwestern University Medical
School
Prentice Women's Hospital
333 East Superior Street
Chicago, Illinois 60611, USA

Scott N MacGregor
Department of Obstetrics and
Gynecology
Evanston Hospital
2650 Ridge Avenue
Evanston, Illinois 60203, USA

Bonnie Michaels
Director, Perinatal and Gynecologic
Nursing
Prentice Women's Hospital
333 East Superior Street
Chicago, Illinois 60611, USA

Dietra Delaplane Millard
Assistant Professor of Pediatrics
Division of Neonatalogy
Prentice Women's Hospital
333 East Superior Street
Chicago, Illinois 60611, USA

Barbara A Morse
Fetal Alcohol Education Program
7 Kent Street
Brookline, Massachusetts 02146,
USA

Melinda Noonan
Perinatal Instructor
Prentice Women's Hospital
333 East Superior Street
Chicago, Illinois 60611, USA

Jane W Schneider
Perinatal Center for Chemical
Dependence
215 East Chicago Avenue
Chicago, Illinois 60611, USA

John J Sciarra
Professor and Chairman
Department of Obstetrics and
Gynecology
Northwestern University Medical
School
333 East Superior Street
Chicago, Illinois 60611, USA

Lyn Weiner
Fetal Alcohol Education Program
7 Kent Street
Brookline, Massachusetts 02146,
USA

Jeanne M Wilton
Lactation Consultant
Prentice Women's Hospital
333 East Superior Street
Chicago, Illinois 60611, USA

Barry Zuckerman
Associate Professor of Pediatrics
Boston University School of
Medicine
Director, Division of
Developmental and Behavioral
Pediatrics
Boston City Hospital
818 Harrison Avenue
Boston, Massachusetts 02118, USA

Introduction
The Interfaces of Perinatal Addiction

Ira J Chasnoff

In the last few years, problems associated with drug use in pregnancy have become endemic. As cocaine has become the drug of choice for millions of Americans, including pregnant women, as AIDS has become more commonly recognized in women and infants, and as legal cases have begun to raise the question of fetal abuse, no professional group has come forward to serve as advocate for this special population of substance abusers. Meanwhile, however, physicians, nurses, social service agencies and public health officials have all been faced with increasing numbers of infants showing the detrimental effects of their mothers' drug use.

Although problems of substance abuse in pregnancy have received increasing attention in the medical literature since the early 1970s, there has recently been a very rapid increase in the number of articles published related to this field. The reasons for this new interest are easily understood when current statistics from the National Institute on Drug Abuse are reviewed[1]. Although patterns of abuse of alcohol, marijuana, heroin and other substances by women of childbearing age have changed very little over the last ten years, the incidence of cocaine use in this special population has been rising rapidly, a reflection of cocaine's increasing popularity among the general population of the United States.

Additionally, our concept of teratology has changed in that we now recognize that, although most drugs of use and abuse do not produce congenital malformations, there are definite behavioral and neurological effects that place the neonate, infant and child at risk for developmental abnormality.

PATTERNS OF DRUG USE

Early studies evaluating drug use by women during pregnancy revealed that around 50-60% of women used some analgesic during pregnancy, and sedative drug use by pregnant women ranged around 25%[2]. The majority of the women involved in studies such as these were women who were receiving prenatal care and were obtaining many of the medications by prescription

1

from their physicians. Use of illicit drugs was rarely considered. During a six-month period in 1982, screening of all women enrolling at Prentice Women's Hospital and Maternity Center for routine prenatal care revealed that 3% of these women had sedative-hypnotics in their urine at the time of admission to the general maternity clinic[3]. This study was performed prior to cocaine's becoming society's drug of choice. Currently, with an estimated 20 million using it on a regular basis[4], the number of pregnant cocaine users in the United States has rapidly risen, but no figures as to the actual prevalence are available.

CHILD ABUSE AND NEGLECT

The risk maternal drug use poses for the child does not end at birth. In New York City, it was estimated that 50% of all child abuse and neglect cases involved drug abuse, and if alcohol was included, substance abuse was involved in 64% of child abuse cases[5]. In a survey conducted by the Child Abuse Prevention Program, Department of Health Services in Los Angeles, California, of a total of 5973 cases of child abuse reported in 1985, 538 cases (9%) involved neonatal withdrawal due to maternal drug use in pregnancy. In the first six months of 1986, 403 of 4299 cases (9.4%) of child abuse were reported due to maternal addiction during pregnancy. The patterns of drug use in this population showed a shift towards a higher frequency of cocaine use among the reported cases in the first six months of 1986 as compared to 1985.

In Illinois in fiscal year 1987, more than 91,000 infants and children were reported to the state child abuse hotline, a 50% increase over fiscal year 1986. Of those reports, 530 were due to the finding of a drug of abuse in a neonate's urine. This represented a 77% increase in such reports over a one-year span. Even so, the majority of cases of maternal substance abuse in pregnancy go undetected and unreported.

A study conducted in 1986 by the Illinois Department of Children and Family Services evaluated a random sample of 385 children who had become wards of the state due to abuse or neglect and who subsequently had been placed in foster care. It was found that about half of these children came from parents or caretakers who were known or suspected substance abusers. These parents were often reluctant to accept help: 55% rejected social services when offered and 68% rejected substance abuse services. In addition, and perhaps most striking, 11% of these children in foster care had had serious medical problems (abstinence, seizures, respiratory distress) at birth related to *in utero* exposure to substances of abuse.

With the current shift to cocaine as one of the most common primary

2

drugs of abuse, polydrug abuse has also become more common, with the majority of cocaine users abusing marijuana and/or alcohol and/or cigarettes in addition. Thus, evaluation of risk factors for the pregnant substance abuser and her newborn must take into consideration the effects of these secondary drugs of abuse. Another mediating factor in the fetus' response to drug exposure is related to the individual's ability to metabolize and tolerate the illicit drug. This ability is determined through a variety of genetic and physiologic factors.

Multiple other factors in the environment of the pregnant substance-abusing woman, including poor nutrition, lack of prenatal care, maternal psychopathology and the drug-seeking lifestyle, affect the ultimate outcome of the passively exposed infant and must be considered in the interpretation of clinical and research information.

SECONDARY DRUG USE

The association between drug or alcohol use and cigarette smoking has been repeatedly observed [6], and the effects of cigarettes on the developing fetus must be considered in any infant being evaluated for intrauterine exposure to drugs of abuse. Smoking women have infants with significantly lower birth weight than non-smoking women; however, no increase in neonatal mortality rate or congenital anomalies have been observed among these infants. Of interest, among the many studies relating smoking and low birth weight, none took into account that smoking itself is associated with heavier alcohol use; this could have contributed a significant portion of the variance in birth weight. Heavy use of additional substances, such as caffeine, further complicates the evaluation of drug effects on the fetus.

AIDS

In a study performed in 1982, prior to the widespread presence of acquired immune deficiency syndrome (AIDS) in the Chicago area, infants born to intravenous drug-using mothers were found to have a more frequent rate of infections than infants of oral drug-abusing mothers or drug-free infants[7]. The number of episodes of illness was also increased among infants of intravenous-addicted mothers. Some of the illnesses were the clinical manifestations resulting from exposure to specific organisms (*Chlamydia*, pneumonia, thrush, monilia diaper rash) while others were caused by a spectrum of micro-organisms (bronchiolitis, otitis media). Of note is the finding that the thrush in these patients was qualitatively different than the

3

thrush usually observed in non-drug-exposed infants. It was more severe and persisted for a longer time than usual despite the use of conventional antifungal therapy. These observations suggested a possible immune defect related to intravenous opiate use. None of these infants developed severe opportunistic infections or acquired immune deficiency syndrome (AIDS).

Recently, exposure to the human immunodeficiency virus (HIV) has become an increasingly important aspect of assessment and management of the newborn delivered to a drug-abusing mother. Women with a history of intravenous drug use, prostitution or sexual intercourse with a bisexual or intravenous drug-using male should be considered at high risk for exposure. Currently, 25% of the intravenous drug-using women enrolled in our program are HIV positive. Almost all infants delivered to HIV antibody positive women will themselves be seropositive at birth, given the ease with which IgG antibodies cross the placenta. The true HIV status of an infant cannot usually be determined until 12 to 15 months of age, by which time all passively acquired maternal antibody should be absent from the infant's serum. Aside from the dysmorphologic and life-threatening infectious complications which have been reported to occur in infants with the acquired immune deficiency syndrome, these infants also exhibit poor growth and developmental delay[8]. Early studies in our program have also demonstrated impairment of mother – infant attachment and interaction, a not surprising consequence of a mother's knowing her child has a potentially fatal illness.

IMPLICATIONS FOR RISK

Little reliable information regarding long-term outcome of infants passively exposed to drugs of abuse is available. To best evaluate these children at school age, environmental factors must be taken into account. These environmental factors are not only socioeconomic but should encompass aspects of the mother – infant relationship, including maternal psychopathology and personality. One study which did attempt to control for the caretaking environment of substance-exposed children compared these infants to those whose families began to use drugs after the birth of the children[9]. No differences were found between the in-utero-exposed children and the children exposed to the social environment of drug-using caretakers. Further studies are needed before final conclusions can be drawn as to the long-term effects of in utero drug exposure on infants and child development.

The problems involved in evaluating the effects of maternal exposure to substances of abuse on the developing fetus and infant are multiple, not the least of which are the difficulties involved in following these infants over a long period of time. The chaotic and transient nature of the drug-seeking environment impairs the intensive follow-up and early intervention processes necessary to insure maximum development by each infant. In addition, most women from substance-abusing backgrounds lack a proper model for parenting. These factors, compounded by the early neurobehavioural deficits of the drug-exposed newborns, earmark these infants to be at high risk for continuing developmental and later school problems.

A key problem in the field of substance abuse in pregnancy is a public and professional lack of knowledge of the subject. Few prospective parents recognize that their lifestyle, especially drug use and abuse, has a powerful impact on the outcome of their newborn infant. Information about the hazards of substance abuse during pregnancy must be presented to the public in a straightforward, non-judgmental manner. In this way, information regarding the effects of any licit or illicit drug use during pregnancy can become part of the public consciousness.

It is easy to overlook the newborn's passive exposure to drugs of abuse, for the assessment of maternal chemical dependence tends to be insufficient in most instances. Currently, pediatricians often must rely on scanty information from the prenatal period when assessing a newborn displaying withdrawal or the neurotoxic effects of drug exposure. A study of alcoholism by Sokol *et al.* found that 'clinicians are continuing to miss the diagnosis in at least three of every four alcohol-abusing patients. It is unlikely that there is any other obstetric diagnosis that is missed as often'[10]. Today, few patients limit their abuse to alcohol and, with the current phenomenon of polydrug abuse, chemical dependence in the pregnant woman with the concomitant effects in the newborn most assuredly is one of the most frequently missed diagnoses in the perinatal period. When an untoward event in the perinatal period does occur, whether it be a perinatal cerebral infarction, unexpected premature delivery or an unexplained accident of pregnancy such as an abruption, maternal substance abuse must be placed in the differential diagnosis. The irritable newborn or one with unusual complications should be assessed with a full historical evaluation for substance exposure and, when indicated, a full toxicologic urine screen. Pediatricians have come to realize that intrauterine drug exposure has become a major cause of perinatal morbidity and mortality, and an area that can no longer be overlooked[11].

The developmental risks imposed by the maternal use of substances of abuse are, perhaps more than many other risk factors, preventable. However, the first step in prevention and intervention relies on the establishment in the medical and public sectors of a perception of risk. This perception should be based on education of the public as to the clear effects maternal substance abuse have on pregnancy and neonatal outcome. Secondly, the medical and psychological communities must begin to better understand risk-taking behavior and the personality and motivational factors that engender and enhance this behavior. We must delineate the measureable outcomes that best express the damage of maternal substance abuse to the child, then use the most effective means of increasing the public's recognition of this risk and influencing the individual's will to act to reduce relevant risk-taking behavior.

This book presents a challenge to its reader to place children and their parents as a priority, to integrate the information from multiple disciplines into a larger field of endeavor and then share this information with others, for health is more than medical care. A child's health relies on the coordination of social, environmental and medical strategies which will ensure the orderly growth and development of that child. Though maternal substance abuse may be a central issue in the life of a child, it is often only a symptom of other facets of lifestyle and environment that must be addressed if a child is to reach his or her full potential.

REFERENCES

1. Clayton, R.R. (1985). In a blizzard or just being snowed. In: Kozel, N.J. and Adams, E.H. (eds.) *Cocaine Use in Pregnancy: Epidemiologic and Clinical Perspective, NIDA Research Monograph 61.* pp. 8–22. (Rockville, MD: U.S. Department of Health and Human Services)
2. Kaul, A.F., Harsfield, J.C., Osathanondh, R. and Ostheimen, G.W. (1978). A retrospective analysis of analgesics and sedative-hypnotics in hospitalized obstetrical and gynecological patients. *Drug Intell. Clin. Phar.*, **12**, 95–99
3. Chasnoff, I.J., Schnoll, S.H., Burns, W.J. and Burns, K. (1984). Maternal substance abuse during pregnancy: Effects on infant development. *Neurobehav. Toxicol. Teratol.*, **6**, 277–280
4. Fishbourne, P.M. (1980). *National Survey on Drug Abuse: Main Findings: 1979.* (Rockville, MD, National Institute on Drug Abuse, 1980. DHHS Publication No. ADMBO-976)
5. Marriott, M. (1987). Child abuse cases swamping New York City's family court. *N.Y. Times,* 11/15/87, p. 17
6. Streissguth, A.P., Barr, H.M., Martin, D.C. and Herman, C. (1980). The effects of maternal alcohol, nicotine and caffeine use during pregnancy on infant development at 8 months. *Alc. Clin. Exp. Res.*, **4**, 152–164
7. Rich, K.C. (1986). Immunologic function and AIDS in drug-exposed infants. In: Chasnoff, I.J. (ed.) *Drug Use in Pregnancy: Mother and Child.* pp. 136–146. (Boston, MTP Press Ltd)
8. Iosub, S., Bamji, M., Stone, R.K., Gromisch, D.S. and Wasserman, E. (1987). More on human immunodeficiency virus embryopathy. *Pediatrics*, **80**, 512–516
9. Wilson, G.W., McCreary, K., Kean, J. and Baxter, J. (1979). The development of preschool children of heroin-addicted mothers: A controlled study. *Pediatrics*, **63**, 135–141
10. Sokol, R.J., Miller, S.I. and Martier, S. (1981). *Preventing Fetal Alcohol Effects: A Practical Guide for the Ob/Gyn Physicians and Nurses.* (Rockville, MD, National Institute on Alcohol Abuse and Alcoholism)
11. Chasnoff, I.J., Burns, K.A. and Burns, W.J. (1987). Cocaine use in pregnancy: Perinatal morbidity and mortality. *Neurobehav. Toxicol. Teratol.*, **9**, 291–293

1

Psychosocial Characteristics of Pregnant Women Addicts in Treatment

Amin N Daghestani

Over the years, the epidemiology of substance use by women has been different from that by men. These differences have often related to social and family considerations more than mere physiological ones. Historically, there were more women addicted to opiates than men before the Harrison Act of 1914. A recent study of national trends of drug use among young adults between the years 1975 and 1986 showed a convergence toward zero of the difference between usage levels of the sexes[1]. The male–female ratio of marijuana use has dropped from 3 to 1 in 1980 to 2 to 1 in 1986. Convergence patterns for methaqualone, LSD, and stimulants have been similarly noted, while cigarette smoking has been consistently higher among females than males in college. As more high school and college women use drugs, the subpopulation of drug abusers of the child-bearing age is correspondingly increasing. Although accurate statistics are lacking, this subpopulation represents now the largest group among women addicts.

Despite the fact that the majority of the literature in alcohol and drug abuse has focused on male users, some authors have looked at women's use of alcohol[2-5], drugs[6,7], or treatment outcomes[8]. Initial studies on pregnant addicts focused on the effects of drug use on pregnancy and were published mainly in obstetrical journals[9-11], while other studies explored primarily the effects of alcohol[12-15] or other drugs[16-18] on the newborn.

Research focusing on the pregnant addict has been scarce. Difficulties in studying this patient population stem from the lack of compliance of those patients with follow-up recommendations as well as from the influence of societal stereotypes which emphasize judgemental or moralistic rather than medical models.

This chapter attempts to describe those characteristics which are common to women addicts who present for treatment, their demographic features, drug-use history, and their social and psychological characteristics. Some treatment implications will also be presented.

CLINICAL PRESENTATIONS

Evaluation of the pregnant addicted patient should be thorough and comprehensive. It should include a detailed history of drug use such as the kind, amount, duration, frequency and route of administration. The level of family support available during the recent crisis sustained by the patient should be assessed. Besides physical and obstetric examination, laboratory work-up should include both urine and blood pregnancy tests as well as toxicological screens. For i.v. drug abusers, additional tests such as the HIV and hepatitis screens should be considered.

As in other drug-abusing populations, pregnant addicts tend to show up late in gestation for the initial intervention. Both the denial of the illness and social stigma associated with it may contribute to this phenomenon. Eventually, it is the apprehension about delivery and the complications of drug usage rather than the use itself which bring the pregnant addict to treatment.

As more women work in traditionally male jobs, their experience of corresponding stress is likewise increasing. Other significant stressors related to child-rearing: living alone, lower income scales, and fewer financial resources. Women drug abusers tend to have more dysfunction in their family of origin and to have partners who are most likely drug dealers or abusers themselves. Psychologically, they present with a higher level of depression, anxiety, sense of powerlessness, and a lower level of self-esteem and self-confidence. The stability which the pregnant women needs is the very same thing which she lacks the most. In addition to the social and physical dysfunctions suffered by the patient, the pregnant addict must deal with the additional sense of guilt and shame of 'hurting' her growing fetus as a result of drug use.

The psychiatric evaluation of the patient reveals the presence of multiple social, family, and interpersonal losses. With a weakened support system and tenuous ego strength, symptoms of anxiety, depression, or suicidal ideations or attempts may be present. Other psychopathology often found includes mood disorders, schizophrenia, and anxiety and phobic disorders. The personality disorders most frequently diagnosed are borderline, passive, aggressive, and antisocial personality disorders. The relationship of psycho-pathology to substance use disorder should be thoroughly assessed in relation to the primary and secondary diagnoses.

In terms of the pregnancy itself, female addicts often tend not to suspect their pregnancy early, sometimes not even until the pregnancy is in its second trimester. The missed menses is interpreted by the addict as a result of drug use and not conception. This is explained by the difficulty these patients have in the level of their self-care. The decreased awareness of bodily changes will

8

make the suspicion of pregnancy by the woman very low. As a result, addicted pregnant women tend to seek help during their third trimester rather than during the first or second one.

Associated medical problems often serve as the primary reason for entry into treatment. Two explanations for this have been entertained: a socio-cultural one, whereby women are more allowed to be medically ill, and a biological predisposition, whereby drugs exert a more toxic influence on women than on men.

Female drug abusers complain of more medical problems than male drug abusers do [19], and it is those medical problems more than the psychological ones which precipitate the woman's entrance into drug-abuse treatment. The medical problems which the female addicts are at increased risk for involve infections, anemia, and sexually-transmitted diseases: gonorrhea, tricho-moniasis, and chlamydia. Other physical problems include menstrual dysfunction[20], decreased fertility, hepatitis, hypertension, adult-onset diabetes and urinary tract infections.

DEMOGRAPHIC ISSUES

The average age of the pregnant addict is estimated to be 24. She tends to have children more often than not. For some, this constitutes a source of additional responsibilities for which these women are not prepared. Mulford[21] found in a sample of female problem drinkers in Iowa that over a fourth of the women felt that their children were critical of their drinking.

Pregnant addicts tend to be poorly educated, although treatment centers are increasingly seeing more educated and professional women on admission. Up until recently, female opiate addicts in treatment came from lower socioeconomic classes and had fewer job opportunities available to them.

Partners of pregnant addicts tend to be substance abusers themselves more than partners of male addicts do. For such a relationship, certain stereotyped images have been described. One of these images recently outlined by Morningstar and Chitwood[22] depicts the female cocaine addict as a 'cocaine whore' in contrast to the gun-toting 'cocaine cowboy' of the male.

DRUG-USE HISTORY

A detailed history of drug use in the pregnant addicted patient reveals a number of similarities to and differences from that noted in the general addicted population. Such a history should examine the kinds of drugs used, the setting of abuse, its duration, frequency and route of administration.

Women, more likely than men, will use socially acceptable drugs and perceive their use of psychoactive substances as a form of coping[23,24]. Patterns of drug use and the type of abused drugs which are socially acceptable, on the other hand, do change from time to time. For the pregnant women, the use of heroin during the 1970s and earlier was being reported in the literature to be more common than any other substances of abuse[25-28]. Reports of other drugs used by pregnant women include marijuana, alcohol and cocaine. Surprisingly, the common perception that women prefer the use of tranquilizers more than other drugs is not substantiated in the literature in regard to the pregnant addict.

Hingson et al.[29] found that those women who were told that they would be tested for drugs reported more marijuana use during pregnancy than did untested women. Urine assays identified more women who used marijuana during pregnancy than were willing to admit it in the interview. Alcohol consumption in pregnant women was recently documented by Mills et al.[30] and Weiner et al.[31]. Cocaine became one of the most popular drugs during the mid-1980s and the majority of pregnant cocaine users continued to use it during pregnancy[32].

Poly-drug use, which often signifies a more advanced pathology, has also been reported in the pregnant woman. Some of the most common combinations include the use of alcohol and cocaine or alcohol, marijuana and tobacco[33].

For most pregnant addicts, drug use was present before the onset of pregnancy and continued into the second or even third trimester before the women appeared for treatment.

Routes of drug administration by the pregnant addict include all forms of oral, smoking, insufflation and intravenous use. It is this last form of use which is the most problematic due to the possibility of transmitting the human immunodeficiency virus (HIV) through the sharing of needles.

Intravenous (i.v.) drug users constitute the second largest group of patients to have developed acquired immunodeficiency syndrome (AIDS) in the United States and Europe, and are emerging as the largest source of heterosexual transmission in both areas[34]. Correspondingly, the prevalence of AIDS among women is likely to increase. It is considered to be the leading cause of death for all women between 25 and 34, which is the most fertile age. In New York, some 80% of the city's 1500 HIV-infected women have taken i.v. drugs or are the sex partners of i.v. drug abusers, and most of the nearly 300 children with AIDS in New York had been infected as a result of i.v. drug use by one or both of their parents[35].

Sexually active female i.v. drug addicts constitute a particularly high-risk group for developing AIDS. They are exposed to the HIV infection through both sexual activity and i.v. drug abuse. The pregnancy rate for this group is

10

high, and the risk for transmitting HIV to infants is increased. Strategies for preventing AIDS must educate women about ways to empower themselves[36].

SOCIAL ISSUES

Pregnant addicts suffer from the same social problems which affect all other women addicts. Criminality, prostitution, and vulnerability to physical abuse are the three main issues here.

The relationship between substance abuse and female criminality was reviewed by James et al.[37] and Martin et al.[38]. Women are often 'used' for drug trafficking because of a lower suspicion index. In one study, half of a group of imprisoned female subjects was found to have used heroin daily[39]. Unlike male drug abusers where the crimes committed involve robbery, burglary, and assault, the crimes committed by female drug abusers involve shoplifting, drug sale and prostitution.

Prostitution for some female drug addicts has the main purpose of obtaining money to support drug usage[40]. These women usually lack necessary social and family support to help them during the period of pregnancy. The men they associate with are often unreliable. The women feel isolated with very limited resources available to them. They are often involved in an abusive relationship. This vulnerability to physical abuse may stem from a history of being abused as children. With successful treatment of the chemical dependency, the prostitution behavior will most likely cease. Such a possibility of emancipation from prostitution to adult stability has been discussed by Renshaw[41].

PSYCHOLOGICAL ISSUES

Pregnancy brings certain unresolved issues for the women to the forefront. This is most evident in those individuals who have not gone through various psychological development tasks successfully. These unresolved issues in the pregnant addict usually center around three major problem areas: (1) difficulties in object relationships, (2) difficulties with body image, and (3) intimacy problems.

Developmentally the pregnant addict is seen as not having experienced her mother as a good, nurturing or supporting figure in her formative years; thus, she does not perceive herself as a potentially 'good' mother. She may have ambivalent feelings regarding her own attitudes toward pregnancy, labor, child rearing, or self-concept and self-esteem[42].

The healthy pregnant woman experiences her pregnancy with joy and

11

fulfillment. For the drug addict, however, the bodily sensations of pregnancy are often interpreted as uncomfortable or dangerous, especially in the woman whose earlier life experiences have not included sufficient care, love or attention. The failure in contraception or the ignorance about its prevention may catch the woman unprepared for pregnancy and impose a sudden demand for an adjustment in lifestyle which she may not succeed in accomplishing.

Problems in interpersonal relationships affect the pregnant addict's interactions with significant people in her life. One individual who becomes the object of conflict is the father of the baby. Factors which affect the pregnant addict's feelings towards this person is his presence or absence and the level of support. Not knowing the identity of the father, as the case might sometimes be, introduces a host of added psychological and social complications.

The pregnant addict may unconsciously use pregnancy to satisfy an unresolved childhood fantasy, as a means of replacing a lost object, or as an adjustment to marital discord.

The pregnancy represents dramatic physical and hormonal change associated with alterations in body image. Such an image has been considered the mediator of basic trust, attachment and human interactions[43]. However, these changes in body image may signal a breakdown of boundaries between self and others, and between inner and outer self[44]. Problems with body image perceptions may be attributed to early disturbances in internalizations of parts of the parents or their attitudes toward their own bodies.

Problems in intimacy are closely related to failure in establishing attachments, and it is this kind of problem which eventually proves to be the most difficult barrier to recovery during the treatment process[45]. The intensity of this deficit plays a role in determining the ability of the mother to form bonding ties with her newborn[46-48].

During a normal pregnancy, both the bodily and psychic economy are concentrated on the task of nurturing the developing fetus. For the drug addict, however, this energy is drawn into the preoccupation with obtaining and using drugs. The pregnant addict develops a deficit in her awareness of the 'reality' of the upcoming childbirth. She is not prepared to experience the first cry of the infant or the first physical contact with it as a joyous moment.

During treatment, it is the responsibility of the therapy and medical staff to teach the mother how to hold her baby and to prepare her for the reunion experience. The goal is to help the mother establish an early mother–infant bond instead of experiencing a sense of estrangement and distance. The quality of the mother–infant relationship should be interactive and reciprocal and not passive or uni-directional. During all subsequent visits, the

12

staff should communicate with the mother about the infant's progress, condition and management, and allow her to ventilate her fears and concerns openly and safely.

TREATMENT CONSIDERATIONS

Current treatment models for chemically dependent patients are based on male-oriented approaches. Treatment facilities are inadequate or are not prepared to deal with the multiple needs of the pregnant addict[49]. Programs should be delivered in a context that is compatible with women's styles and orientation, safe from exploitation, and which takes into account women's roles in our society[50]. One particular impediment to an effective therapy program is the attitude of the staff toward the addicted pregnant woman in treatment[51].

Hollstedt et al.[52] described the treatment of fertile-age alcoholics while Marsh et al.[53] described the treatment of female substance abusers, and although Rosett et al.[54] and Singh[55] highlighted their experience in treating the pregnant problem drinkers, few studies have examined thoroughly long-term treatment outcome[56,57].

The comprehensive treatment program should address all complex and special needs of the pregnant addict[58]. Its treatment modalities should include inpatient and outpatient services, as well as provisions for individual, group, family, art and recreational therapies. Its staff should be fully trained in all aspects needed in working with pregnant drug abusers.

Diagnosis and management of the patient with a dual diagnosis, especially the psychotic patient, should be instituted early. A psychiatrist who is trained in the field of substance abuse plays an important role in a team of physicians which include a pediatrician, an obstetrician and a internist[59]. Other needed services should address vocational and skill training, family counseling and legal assistance[60].

Finally, the long-term goals of therapy should deal with those underlying psychological issues related to intimacy and sexuality which, if left undealt with, may place the patient in a vulnerable position for relapse. It is long-term intensive follow-up and active involvement in self-help groups which eventually prove to be the most challenging, yet most important, aspects of working with this patient population.

REFERENCES

1. Johnston, L.D., O'Malley, P.M. and Bachman, J.G. (1987). *National Trends in Drug Use and Related Factors among American High School Students and Young Adults, 1975–1986.* (Rockville, Maryland: National Institute on Drug Abuse)
2. Lindbeck, V.L. (1972). The woman alcoholic: a review of the literature. *Int. J. Addict.,* **7**, 567–80
3. Gomberg, E.S. (1980). Risk factors. In *Alcohol and Women.* (Washington, D.C.:NIAAA)
4. Wilsnack, S.C. and Beckman, L.J. (eds.) (1984). *Alcohol Problems in Women.* (New York: Guildford)
5. Corrigan, E.M. (1980). *Alcoholic Women in Treatment.* (New York: Oxford Press)
6. Sutker, P.B., Archer, R.P. and Allain, A.N. (1978). Drug abuse patterns, personality characteristics and relationships with sex, race, and sensation seeking. *J. Consult. Clin. Psychol.,* **46**, 1374–8
7. Prather, J.E. and Fidell, L.S. (1978). Drug Use and abuse among women: An overview. *Int. J. Addict.,* **13**, 863–5
8. Haver, B. (1987). Female alcoholics. III. Patterns of consumption 3–10 years after treatment. *Acta Psychiatr. Scand.,* **75**, 397–404
9. Neuberg, R. (1970). Drug dependence and pregnancy: A review of the problems and their management. *Br. J. Obstet. Gynaecol.,* **77**, 1117–22
10. Stern, R. (1966). The pregnant addict: A study of 66 case histories, 1950-1959. *Am. J. Obstet. Gynecol.,* **94**, 253–7
11. Blinick, G., Walloch, R., Jerez, E. and Ackerman, B. (1976). Drug addiction in pregnancy and the neonate. *Am. J. Obstet. Gynecol.,* **125**, 135–42
12. Fisher, S.E., Atkinson, M., Burnap, J.K. and Jacobson, S. (1982). Ethanol-associated selective fetal malnutrition: A contributing factor in the fetal alcohol syndrome. *Alcoholism,* **6**, 197–201
13. Sokol, R.J. (1987). Alcohol and abnormal outcomes of pregnancy. *Can. Med. Assoc. J.,* **125**, 143–8
14. Alpert, J.J., Day, N., Dooling, E. and Hingson, R. (1981). Maternal alcohol consumption and newborn assessment: Methodology of the Boston City Hospital Prospective Study. *Neurobehavior. Toxicol. Teratol.,* **3**, 195–200
15. Rosett, H.L. (1984). *Alcohol and the Fetus: A Clinical Perspective.* (New York: Oxford University Press)
16. Woods, J.R., Plessinger, M.A. and Clark, K.E. (1987). Effects of cocaine on uterine blood flow and fetal oxygenation. *J. Am. Med. Assoc.,* **257**, 957–61
17. National Institute on Drug Abuse. (1985). *Consequences of Maternal Drug Abuse. NIDA Research Monograph Series 59.* (Washington, D.C.: National Institute on Drug Abuse).
18. Forfar, J.O. and Nelson, N.M. (1973). Epidemiology of drugs taken by pregnant women - Drugs that may affect the fetus adversely. *Clin. Pharmacol. Ther.,* **14**, 632–42
19. Mondanaro, J. (1981). Medical services for drug dependent women. In Beschner, G.M., Reed, B.G. and Mondanaro, J. (eds.) *Treatment Services for Drug Dependent Women,* Vol. 1. (Rockville, Maryland: NIDA)
20. Wallach, R., Jerez, E. and Blinik, G. (1969). Pregnancy and menstrual functions in narcotic addicts treated with methadone. *Am. J. Obstet. Gynecol.,* **105**, 1226–9
21. Mulford, H.A. (1977). Women and men problem drinkers: Sex differences in patients served by Iowa's community alcoholism centers. *J. Stud. Alcohol,* **38**, 1624–39
22. Morningstar, P. and Chitwood, D.C. (1987). How women and men get cocaine: Sex, role stereotypes and acquisition patterns. *J. Psychoactive Drugs,* **19**, 135–42
23. Reed, B.G. (1985). Drug misuse and dependency in women: The meaning and implications of being considered a special population or a minority group. *Int. J. Addict.,* **20**, 13–62
24. Carr, J. (1975). Drug patterns among drug addicted mothers. *Pediatr. Ann.,* **66**, 409–17
25. Stone, M. (1971). Narcotic addiction in pregnancy. *Am. J. Obstet. Gynecol.,* **109**, 716–23
26. Stotzer, D. and Wardell, J. (1972). Heroin addiction during pregnancy. *Am. J. Obstet. Gynecol.,* **113**, 273–8

27. Yacavone, D. (1976). Heroin addiction, methadone maintenance and pregnancy. *J. Am. Osteopath. Assoc.*, **15**, 826–9
28. Kraus, S. (1958). Heroin addiction among pregnant women and their newborn babies. *Am. J. Obstet. Gynecol.*, **75**, 754–8
29. Hingson, R., Zuckerman, B., Amaro, H., Frank, D.A. and Kayne, H. (1986). Maternal marijuana and neonatal outcome: Uncertainty posed by self-reports. *Am. J. Public Health*, **76**, 667–9
30. Mills, J.L., Graubard, B.I., Harley, E.E., Rhoads, G.G. and Berebdes, H.W. (1984). Maternal alcohol consumption and birth weight. *J. Am. Med. Assoc.*, **255**, 1875–9
31. Weiner, L., Rosett, H.L., Edelin, K.C., Alpert, J.J. and Zuckerman, B. (1983). Alcohol consumption by pregnant women. *Obstet. Gynecol.*, **1**, 6–12
32. Gold, M.S. (1988). The cocaine epidemic in 1988. *The Psychiatric Times*, Feb. 1988, p.6
33. Gibson, G.T., Baghurst, P.A. and Colby, D.P. (1983). Maternal alcohol, tobacco, and cannabis consumption and the outcome of pregnancy. *Aust. NZ J. Obstet. Gynecol.*, **23**, 15–9
34. DesJarlais, D.C. and Friedman, S.R. (1987). HIV infection among intravenous drug users: Epidemiology and risk infection. *AIDS*, **1**, 67–76
35. *American Medical News*, March 18, 1988, p.9
36. Mondanaro, J. (1987). Strategies for AIDS prevention: Motivating health behavior in drug dependent women. *J. Psychoactive Drugs*, **19**, 143–9
37. James, J., Gosho, C. and Watson, R. (1979). The relationship between female criminality and drug use. *Int. J. Addict.*, **14**, 215–29
38. Martin, R.L., Cloninger, C.R. and Guze, S.B. (1982). Alcoholism and female criminality. *J. Clin. Psychiatr.*, **43**, 400–3
39. Sanches, J.E. and Johnson, B.D. (1987). Women and the drug–crime connection: Crime rates among drug abusing women at Rickers Island. *J. Psychoactive Drugs*, **1**, 205–16
40. James, J. (1976). Prostitution and addiction: An interdisciplinary approach. *Addict. Dis.*, **2**, 601–18
41. Renshaw, D.C. (1987). Emancipation: Teen prostitutes to stable adults? *Proc. Inst. Med. Chicago*, **40**, 129–32
42. Gossop, M. (1976). Drug dependence and self-esteem. *Int. J. Addict.*, **11**, 741–53
43. VanderVelde, C.D. (1985). Body in ages of one's self and of others: Developmental and clinical significance. *Am. J. Psychiatr.*, **142**, 527–37
44. Young, I.M. (1984). Pregnant embodiment: Subjectivity and alienation. *J. Med. Phil.*, **9**, 45–62
45. Mondanaro, J., Wedenoja, M., Densen-Gerber, J., Elahi, J., Mason, M. and Redmond, A. (1982). Sexuality and fear of intimacy as barriers to recovery for drug dependent women. In Reed, B.G., Beschner, G.M. and Mondanaro, J. (eds.) *Treatment Series for Drug Dependent Women*, Vol.II. (Rockville, Maryland: NIDA)
46. Klaus, M.H. and Kennell, J.H. (1976). *Maternal–Infant Bonding* (St. Louis: Morley)
47. Coppolino, H.P. (1975). Drug impediments to mothering behavior. *Addict. Dis.*, **2**, 201–8
48. Controneo, M. and Kramer, B.P. (1976). Addiction, alienation and parenting. *Nurs. Clin. N. Am.*, **11**, 517–25
49. Reed, B.G. (1987). Developing women-sensitive drug dependence treatment services, why so difficult? *J. Psychoactive Drugs*, **19**, 151–64
50. Jessup, M. and Green, J.R. 91987). Treatment of the pregnant alcohol-dependent. *J. Psychoactive Drugs*, **19**, 193–203
51. Levy, S.J. and Doyle, K.M. (1974). Attitudes towards women in drug abuse treatment programs. *J. Drug Iss.*, **4**, 428–34
52. Hollstedt, C., Dahlgren, L. and Rydberd, V.C. (1983). Alcoholic women in fertile age treated at an alcoholic clinic. *Acta Psychiatr. Scand.*, **67**, 192–204
53. Marsh, J.C. and Miller, W.A. (1985). Female clients in substance abuse treatment. *Int. J. Addict.*, **20**, 995–1019
54. Rosett, H.L., Weiner, L. and Edelin, K.C. (1983). Treatment experience with pregnant problem drinkers. *J. Am. Med. Assoc.*, **249**, 2029–33

55. Singh, R.K. (1983). Experience with pregnant problem drinkers. *J. Am. Med. Assoc.*, **250**, 2287
56. Suffet, F., Bryce-Buchanan, C. and Brotman, R. (1981). Pregnant addicts in a comprehensive care program: Results of a follow-up survey. *Am. J. Orthopsychiatr.*, **51**, 297–306
57. Suffet, F. and Brotman, R. (1984). A comprehensive care program for pregnant addicts: Obstetrical, neonatal, and child development outcomes. *Int. J. Addict.*, **19**, 199–219
58. Finnegan, L.P. (1978). Drug dependency in pregnancy: Clinical management of mother and child. *Research Monograph Series*. (Rockville, MD: NIDA)
59. Spielvogel, A. and Wile, J. (1986). Treatment of the psychotic pregnant patient. *Psychosomatics*, **27**, 487–92
60. Nelson, L.J. and Milliken, N. (1988). Compelled medical treatment of pregnant women. *J. Am. Med. Assoc.*, **259**, 1060–6

2

Drug Abuse in Pregnancy

Louis G Keith, Scott N MacGregor and John J Sciarra

INTRODUCTION

In 1822 the English writer Thomas de Quincey observed that addiction to opiates (narcomania) not only provided an elevation of the senses and a flight of the imagination, but also offered the 'Keys to Paradise'[1]. Subsequently, other writers have been less enthusiastic about the benefits of addictive substances, especially if used during pregnancy[2]. Alcohol has been held in particular disregard. Between the early 1800's and 1970, a vast literature developed alluding to the detrimental effects of alcohol on pregnancy. No specific set of adverse perinatal outcomes were identified in association with its use until 1968 when Lemoine and co-workers described the now well-accepted stigmata of the Fetal Alcohol Syndrome[3]. Shortly thereafter, their findings were confirmed in two reports by Jones et al.[4,5]. Along with information about the adverse fetal effects of the drug, Thalidomide, these latter two papers undoubtedly contributed to the creation of a favorable climate for the scientific study of the interactions of drugs and pregnancy[6].

Unfortunately, the vast majority of the agents studied have been licit pharmacologic preparations available to pregnant women either by physician prescription or by over-the-counter purchase. By comparison, research into illicit substances has lagged far behind. To date, the bulk of investigations into licit substances with addictive properties (e.g. barbituates, hypnotics, amphetamines, benzodiazepines) have primarily been concerned with teratogenic effects[6] rather than adverse obstetrics or perinatal outcomes[7,8], or the effect on reproduction[9]. In contrast, clinical research on illicit substances used in pregnancy (primarily heroin and cocaine) has been concerned almost exclusively with obstetric and neonatal outcomes rather than teratogenic effects[10-14]. Only recently has it been proposed that the use of cocaine in pregnancy may lead to an increased incidence of fetal anomalies[15]. Notwithstanding this difference, existing information on the obstetric as well as the neonatal effects of addiction to illicit substances in pregnancy is far from complete. To date, no specific syndromes have been

17

described as a result of the use of heroin, cocaine or, for that matter, marijuana, during pregnancy.

Whereas in the past the maternal/fetal problems of heroin addiction were primarily observed in members of the so-called 'underclass', the phenomenon of polydrug abuse and cocaine addiction has spread to the 'middle and upper classes' in the last decade. Moreover, obstetricians commonly encounter patients who inform them (in response to appropriate questions) of their use of sedatives and hypnotics at night, amphetamines in the morning or benzodiazepine derivatives throughout the day. One recent survey of clinicians revealed that they were not only aware of their patients drug-seeking behaviors but wanted to become more involved in helping them counteract this activity. These physicians maintained their attitudes despite recognition of the illicit nature of the abused substances.

The purpose of this chapter is to review current knowledge regarding pregnancy, the addictive process, and perinatal outcome. Our focus will be the effects of opiates and cocaine, although appropriate reference will be made to other substances. Readers with particular interest in the effects of alcohol abuse during pregnancy may consult references 2 and 16–21. Clinical experience obtained at the Northwestern Memorial Hospital Perinatal Center for Chemical Dependence (PCCD) will be referred to extensively throughout the chapter.

ADDICTION IN PREGNANCY

General Comments

Whereas widespread use of prescription medications and over-the-counter remedies during pregnancy is common and well documented[22], the incidence of addiction to illicit drugs in pregnancy is unknown. In all likelihood, it remains relatively low in most small to medium sized communities or in semi-rural areas, but in some large urban centers it may reach serious proportions and account for considerable numbers of adverse maternal and neonatal outcomes[23–26].

Recent studies have attempted to evaluate prevalence of cocaine use in the United States. According to one survey published in 1983, cocaine use quadrupled among college age adults in the decade between 1972 and 1982[27]. Thirty-three million individuals were thought to be affected. A second, smaller survey of 50,000 women showed that women between 18 and 34 years of age constituted 15% of regular cocaine users[28]. These data suggest that cocaine use among pregnant women has become increasingly common.

The Addictive Life Style

The addictive life style is not conducive to maternal and fetal health/well being. The mother's life generally is in a state of disarray, often to the point of being chaotic. Dysfunctional behavior patterns involving the family of origin or the marital consort occur commonly, even though the husbands and/or biologic fathers of the children of addicted women may not personally abuse drugs. The drug-seeking patient often relates a history of parental substance abuse and dysfunctional family-of-origin relationships[29].

Specific Problems

Several problems are commonly associated with addiction complicating pregnancy. These include but are not limited to the following:

(a) **Legal Entanglements.** Whereas alcohol may be purchased legally, the use of heroin, cocaine or other illicit substances carries a serious risk of indictment, incarceration or both because of the illegal status afforded these agents. Attempts to control, reduce or eliminate addiction frequently are undertaken only in response to court orders or in the hope that such activity will be looked upon with favor by law enforcement agencies.

(b) **Poor Compliance with Medical Protocols.** The constant and recurring need to self medicate may interfere with regular clinic attendance. Unless the patient is enrolled in a highly structured program with a well-developed follow-up component, poor or non-existant care is the rule[24,26]. The total number of prenatal visits *per se* (Table 2.1) may be misleading, and the numbers of 'no-show clinic appointments' are more revealing of the extent of non-compliance. For example, between July 1, 1986 and June 30, 1987 the 'no-show' rate averaged 38% at the obstetric clinic of the PCCD. The majority of the patients seen during this period had cocaine addictions. This figure appears considerably higher than the rates observed when the preponderance of patients were addicted to opiates. The 'no-show' rate takes on greater significance when it is recognized that patients actively addicted to cocaine frequently are given more appointments because of their inherent medical risks.

Table 2.1 Prenatal visits, 1982–86, by class of addiction, Northwestern Memorial Hospital, Chicago

Type	Mean	SD
Controls	10.2	3.7
All drug patients		
Cocaine (C)	8.4	4.3
Opiates (O)	8.6	5.6
C & O	7.3	4.7
Others	9.9	4.5

(c)   **Poor Nutrition and Health**. The nutritional status of addicts varies widely. Based upon the degree and length of the addiction (rather than the specific substance of abuse), desire to eat may be substantially reduced. Marked anemia and hidden mineralogic deficits may exist at the onset of pregnancy. Poor dentition, as well as the abdominal discomfort associated with chronic alcoholic gastritis or the gastrointestinal side effects of opiate use, contribute to inadequate caloric intake. For the cocaine-abusing individual, the most intense and sensual gastronomic delights pale in comparison with the anticipated pleasure afforded by her substance of abuse.

(d)   **Variations in drugs ingested**. Neither the addict nor her physician can discern the quantity of pharmacologically active agents in street drugs nor the extent to which they may have been adulterated. This statement holds true for heroin used for injection, skin popping or snorting, as well as for cocaine used for inhalation or free-basing and 'crack', the smokeable variation of cocaine. In the latter instance the end product of the basic distillation process may vary somewhat based upon the quality of the cocaine originally used in the chemical transformation process.

(e)   **Switching of drugs**. Only a modest percentage of addicts abuse one substance to the exclusion of all others. Even the so-called 'innocuous' addiction of tobacco often is accompanied by liberal use of alcohol and vice-versa. Depending on daily street availability, addicts tend to 'switch' drugs, either intraclass (opiates and heroin to CNS depressants such as barbituates) or interclass (opiates to CNS stimulants such as cocaine). The length of abuse of specific substances depends as much upon substance availability as it does upon idiosyncratic reactions of patients which demand a change.

(f) **Combined drug effects.** Poly-drug abuse has been particularly prevalent since the early 1980s[13]. It is common to obtain 4–5 responses to a substance abuse survey regardless of whether the questions pertain to 'present use' or 'ever used' agents. Exclusive of tobacco and alcohol, only about 24% of pregnant respondants queried at the PCCD between 1982 and 1986 stated that they abused a single substance to the exclusion of all others.

Financial Considerations

The financial basis for the reimbursement of medical care for addicted pregnant women is problematic. Only rarely are all costs covered by third parties. Rarer still is the patient who assumes responsibility for her own health care expenses. Most often than not, patients from the middle and lower classes are able to obtain state-subsidized health care benefits on the basis of their pregnant condition, but governmental plans rarely reimburse the totality of costs, especially if the patient is enrolled in a program that provides psychosocial counseling and pediatric follow-up, in addition to prenatal care.

If payment for health care is considered problematic in the mind of the addicted individual, payment for substances of abuse is usually not. All too frequently, perversion of available personal resources sets in motion the train of events leading to ill health and in many instances, criminal behavior. It is widely appreciated that a full blown heroin or cocaine habit may require the expenditure of $200–400/day. In contrast, alcohol may cost only $20–25/day and pill habits even less. Regardless, the question of the source of these funds is valid especially if the woman is unemployed or unmarried. The first available resource is family funds. When these are exhausted, other sources may be found. The drain on family funds often initiates neglect and abuse of existing family members, especially children whose nutrition may be first to suffer. Petty thievery, shoplifting, drug dealing and prostitution all may play a part later unless the patient's male partner assumes this responsibility in return for the woman's companionship, sexual favors or both. Even when such 'sponsorship' takes place, the patient is often poorly motivated to use her available resources to provide adequately for her physical needs or those of her family.

ADDICTION AS A MANIFESTATION OF DYSFUNCTION

Rarely does addiction manifest itself for the first time during pregnancy. While many obstetricians can recognize signs of addiction in their patients, few are prepared to assume the dual role of obstetrician and psychotherapist. This is not to say that obstetricians cannot or should not make appropriate comments and give good advice regarding the health benefits of the elimination of substances of abuse. Rather, they must recognize that the process of addiction began prior to pregnancy within the family of origin[30,31], and that long-term psychosocial intervention is necessary not only during pregnancy but after as well.

Drugs of Addictive Power

Drug histories ideally should be obtained as a longitudinal survey beginning in early adolescence. Starting with tobacco and alcohol, use of each specific substance of abuse should be added and the age of initiation of use indicated. For the months preceeding the last normal known menstrual period, a detailed monthly assessment of drug use should be obtained for licit as well as illicit drugs. This assessment then can be recorded throughout pregnancy. Methods such as these are more likely to expose the full range of substances abused and deliniate the extent of need for psychosocial guidance and intervention during and after pregnancy.

With rare exception, substances abused during pregnancy are those abused when the individual was in the non-pregnant state. Exceptions relate to the specific idiosyncrasies of pregnancy. A woman may shy away from agents which accentuate her nausea or upset her gastrointestinal tract and replace these drugs with others which have the same general effect, absent the gastrointestinal upset.

The Effects of Addiction on Menstruation and Reproductive Potential

Depending to some extent on the agent of abuse, menstrual abnormalities are relatively common in substance-abusing women. Amenorrhea is reported more frequently than hypermenorrhea[32,33]. Amenorrhea is most commonly associated with heroin addiction, although it may also be observed in women using methadone[32] or chronically addicted to cocaine. The true frequency and duration of amenorrhea in women addicted to cocaine is unknown, because they are not regular seekers of health care except in crisis situations and the veracity of their medical histories cannot be relied upon. Recently, a

36-year-old grandmother who was chronically addicted to cocaine presented for the first time to the PCCD in the advanced stages of pregnancy. She stated that she had been amenorrheic for so long that she no longer considered the possibility of getting pregnant. Histories such as these previously were confined almost exclusively to opiate addicts. Menstrual periodicity is not affected adversely by alcoholism.

The effects of all substances of addictive power upon the hypothalamic–pituitary–ovarian axis have not yet been clarified[9]. However, impaired fertility may exist for at least two reasons: (1) menstrual irregularity, oligo-ovulation and decreased libido associated with chronic opiate abuse; (2) impairment of tubal function secondary to salpingitis from acquired sexually transmitted diseases. This latter consideration is especially prominent if the patient has multiple sexual partners, if the patient has prostituted herself or if her partner has prostituted himself to support one or both addictions. In 1975, it was proposed that methadone may stimulate ovulation and lead to multiple births[34]. However, this isolated observation has not been confirmed in other studies. Unfortunately, the problems inherent in following addictive lifestyles are so complex as to make it unlikely in the foreseeable future that broad-based population studies will be able to generate definitive answers to questions regarding fertility rates for addicted women.

Perinatal Pharmacology

Prior to examining the effects of drug use during pregnancy, it is necessary to discuss perinatal pharmacology. The mother, the placenta and the fetus each exert some action on the metabolism of ingested drugs and thereby influence the total effect. For example, the route of administration of a drug influences its ability to cross the placenta. Oral administration may reduce the drug's ability to cross the placenta if significant first-pass metabolism occurs in the liver. In contrast, drugs taken intravenously, intranasaly or by inhalation may more readily cross the placenta since these routes avoid first-pass metabolism. In addition, pregnancy *per se* may alter drug metabolism, leading either to diminished or enhanced drug effects. Since plasma and liver cholinesterase activity are decreased during pregnancy, the metabolism of agents such as cocaine is also diminished. Such alteration in maternal metabolism may enhance both maternal and fetal drug effects.

All drugs cross the placenta to some extent. Several factors enhance the ability of drugs to cross the placenta. In particular, lipid solubility and low molecular weight (<1000) are important. In general, any drug which crosses the blood–brain barrier and exerts an effect on the central nervous system, such as opiates, alcohol and cocaine, will readily cross the placenta.

Additional factors which influence the ability of drugs to cross the placenta include: protein-binding capacity of the drug (only the unbound form crosses), serum pH and the ionization state of the drug (the non-ionized form crosses more readily).

The fetus is particularly susceptible to potentially teratogenic effects of drugs during the first eight weeks of pregnancy[35]. This period is critical for normal embryonic development. Drugs which have teratogenic potential should be avoided during this period. Unfortunately, all too often women are unaware that they are pregnant during the first few weeks of embryonic life. Not all embryos exposed to teratogenic drugs, such as alcohol and possibly cocaine, develop problems. Therefore, the fetus must have some level of genetic susceptibility to the effects of the drug. Relatively little is known about the disposition and metabolism of drugs in the fetus. Clearly, the fetus and placenta metabolize some drugs; however, immaturity of developing organs may result in failure to observe all the biologic effects.

MANAGEMENT OF THE PREGNANCY/ADDICTION COMPLEX

Basic Service Organization

Depending upon the study reviewed and the year of its publication, as many as 50–60% of addicts receive no prenatal care whatsoever[24,26]. It is not possible to state to what extent these figures are reliable for women giving birth in the decade between 1975 and 1985 when polydrug and cocaine abuse have become more common. Regardless of the extent of underutilization of existing services, providing basic prenatal care to addicted women is inherently more difficult, requires more skilled personel and is considerably more costly than providing care to other patients.

A team approach is required, and the team should be comprised of experienced individuals who participate because of their desire to do so. Ambivalent service providers who care for addicted parturients will be discouraged easily and early. A comprehensive care team should include, at the minimum, individuals from the following disciplines:

(a)   nurses experienced in offering pregnancy support and health counseling to addicted women;
(b)   obstetricians experienced in treating the general medical problems of addicted parturients;
(c)   maternal–fetal medicine specialists capable of treating the high-risk aspects of addicted women (especially those addicted to cocaine);

(d)   clinical psychologists to provide individual or group psychosocial therapy;

(e)   behavioral psychologists capable of assessing the degrees of social maladjustment exhibited by patients;

(f)   social workers to assist in the development of appropriate contacts with assisting agencies.

Although members of the team may function individually, their efforts must be integrated and directed toward a common goal. Team members should meet regularly to review the status of all patients. Obstetricians should not direct methadone doses or other aspects of drug management, detoxification or withdrawal. Similarly, psychologists, psychiatrists and social workers should not direct obstetric decisions. Each member of the team should provide care commensurate with his/her area of expertise. Such an approach helps negate attempts of the addict to 'split' staff opinions and goals or manipulate individual team members in order to secure favors or placate perceived needs. Uniformity of care and consistency in decision making processes is more likely to occur when the team acts as a firm and cohesive unit.

The goals of therapy should extend beyond the pregnancy and be directed at long-term rehabilitation as well. To assist in this process the patient should see the same team members consistently. By becoming acquainted with those responsible for her prenatal care and establishing trust and open lines of communication with them, the patient is more likely to recognize the importance of her participation in the health care process.

Supporting Services

At a minimum, the following support services should be available:

(a)   inpatient hospitalization service on a chemical dependency unit for detoxification as needed;

(b)   financial services to assist meeting basic living needs;

(c)   dietetic services to provide information about proper nutrition;

(d)   HIV testing and counseling for all patients with individual or partner (past or present) history of i.v. drug use as well as those who have had sexual contact with bisexual males or resorted to prostitution to support their habits;

(e)   pregnancy termination services for HIV-positive patients and others who elect this option;

(f)   visiting nurse services to aid in preparations for the newborn and to supervise ongoing care of the infant postpartum;

(g)   contraceptive counseling services to offer information in the immediate and late postpartum period;

(h)   pediatric liaisons for immediate evaluation of the newborn for the presence of drugs, HIV antibody, withdrawal symptoms, risk of sudden infant death syndrome (SIDS) and other perinatal risk factors;

(i)   developmental follow-up clinics to assess the infant's progress.

Ideally, support services should be coordinated by various members of the health care team. Since many addicted parturients often show little or no personal responsibility for problem solving, ready access is the key to utilization of all support services.

Protocols for Prenatal Care

Adequate prenatal care begins with a thorough medical evaluation and appropriate laboratory studies. Maternal urine ideally should be obtained at each visit and screened for the presence of illicit drugs. Routine parameters for evaluation of fetal well being should be employed throughout the pregnancy. Intrauterine growth retardation should always be considered in addicted parturients[10,12]. Table 2.2 is derived from our 1986–87 requisite laboratory examination list; the times for their repetition (when required) are noted.

Maternal infection must be treated aggressively. This is especially true of urinary tract infections, vaginitis, and venereal disease. Tuberculosis, when first identified during pregnancy by a positive skin test, should be evaluated by a chest X-ray with shielded abdomen. If a VDRL test is positive, a fluorescent treponenmal antibody absorption (FTA-ABS) test should also be performed. Treatment should be undertaken *only* if the latter test is reactive and no prior treatment has been administered, as drug addiction itself may be associated with a weakly positive VDRL test or, for that matter, a false positive Elisa test for HIV.

Liberal utilization of ultrasound is advised. Gestational age should be established and fetal growth patterns documented by serial examinations. A growth adjusted sonar fetal age (GASA)[36] may be particularly valuable, because accurate menstrual records often are unavailable, and menstrual irregularity is common among opiate addicts. Non-stress testing is advisable weekly from the 32nd week if intrauterine growth retardation (IUGR) is suspected or if the patient abuses cocaine.

Table 2.2 Perinatal Center for Chemical Dependence – chemical dependency checklist

	Initial visit	15–19 weeks	26–28 weeks	30–34 weeks	36 weeks	41 weeks
Date						
Gest. age						
CBC	X					
HCT					X	
Type & RH	X					
Antibody screen	X					
Serology	X					
Rubella	X					
HGB electrophoresis	X					
Hepatitis profile	X					
UA	X		X			
GC culture	X					
Chlamydia	X					
Pap smear	X					
MSAFP		X				
1° PPBS			X			
HIV (HTLV-III) AB	X		X		X	
US (dating)	X					
US (level II)		X (20–24 wks)				
US (growth)				X (+neurobehav.)		
US (AFV)						X
Nutrition	X					
3 random U/A toxic	X		X		X	
Psychological eval.	X					
Lamaze instruction		Yes No				

Ultrasound for dating can be obtained at either 8–12 weeks (CRL) or 14–24 weeks (BPD/FL) depending on gestational age at initial visit
Circle X when test complete

Name
ID

Table 2.3 Medical complications of addicted patients

Anemia	Phlebitis
Bacteremia	Pneumonia
Cardiac disease,	Septicemia
especially endocarditis	Urinary tract infections
Cellulitis	Cystitis
Cerebrovascular accidents	Urethritis
Poor dental hygiene	Pyelonephritis
Diabetes mellitus	Condyloma acuminatum
Hepatitis - acute/chronic	Gonorrhea
Hypertension	Herpes
Myocardial ischaemia and infarction	Syphilis

Tables 2.3 and 2.4 list some of the medical and obstetric complications traditionally encountered in pregnant heroin and cocaine addicts. It is not possible to state with certainty which conditions related to the addictive process *per se* or to the addictive life style. It also is not possible to discern the relative risk of developing one or more of the associated conditions. Nonetheless, it is becoming increasingly apparent that the unique vaso-constrictive properties of cocaine predispose to early and midtrimester pregnancy losses as well as abruptio placentae, premature rupture of the membranes, diminished fetal growth and congenital anomalies[11,13]. In addition, myometrial stimulant properties of cocaine may be associated with premature labor. Frequently, the onset of these complications is directly related to the last self administration of cocaine. This is particularly relevant for midtrimester bleeding and cramping following prolonged cocaine use. Immediate in-hospital evaluation is required to assess the nature of many of these events.

Table 2.4 Obstetrical complications of addicted patients

Abortion	Intrauterine death
Abruptio placenta	Intrauterine growth retardation
Amnionitis	Placental insufficiency
Breech presentation	Post-partum hemorrhage
Previous C-section	Pre-eclampsia
Chorioamnionitis	Preterm labor
Eclampsia	Premature rupture of membranes
Gestational diabetes	Septic thrombophlebitis

Nutrition

Inadequate nutrition is common among addicted individuals. According to Zuspan and Rayburn[37], a diet containing 100 g of protein per day is beneficial for the pregnant addict. However, this ideal seldom is achieved, despite repetitive counseling by staff and nutritionists. Among the patients studied by these investigators, average protein intakes of less than 50 g/day were common[37].

Supplemental vitamins should be prescribed routinely. In addition to all-purpose prenatal supplements, iron, in the form of ferrous sulfate or gluconate, 300 mg BID or TID, should be given to meet increased needs and counteract pre-existing iron deficiency. Among 137 substance abusing parturients studied at the PCCD between 1982 and 1986, 15, or 11%, had hemoglobins of ≤ 10 g at their initial visits compared to 2 of 123 controls

$(2\%)^{13}$. Zuspan and Rayburn[37] observed that more than 60% (64) of 106 pregnant addicts had abnormally low folic acid levels ($\leq$2.6 mg/dl) and proposed that a test for serum folates be applied routinely to pregnant addicts. Oral folic acid supplementation should be prescribed for individuals with low folate values as well as those with multiple gestations.

Drug Screening

Each pregnant addict ideally should have a urine toxicology screening at every prenatal visit. Unfortunately, many practitioners do not have facilities to perform such examinations on a routine basis except by shipping frozen urine samples to a distant laboratory. As a result, numerous programs and individual physicians have had to forgo screening examinations and rely on patient history. Unfortunately, patient histories are notoriously inaccurate and contribute to the clinical difficulty of providing quality care to addicted individuals. Not only are the quantities of substances consumed highly suspect, but the quality of the agent is also unknown. The same may be said for the adulterants or cutting agents.

Recently, we used prototype screening cards to test for metabolites of marijuana and cocaine. Discarded urine samples were obtained from prenatal patients in the outpatient department and in the labor and delivery suites of Prentice Women's Hospital and Maternity Center, and at the time of the first prenatal examination in a busy private practice. Results were available in minutes, and the technologic requirements to perform the test were truly minimal[38]. As expected, the highest prevalence of 'dirty' urines were collected in the PCCD. Indeed 31% and 34% of samples were positive for metabolites of cocaine and marijuana, respectively. Of interest, the percentage of samples positive for marijuana and cocaine was 19% and 6%, respectively, at the private office.

The routine application of simple screening tests should greatly enhance the clinicians' ability to confront the patient directly about her drug relapses, as far as the specific substances tested. Assuming a cost of $10 per visit for two metabolites at each of 8–10 visits during the course of prenatal care, the total expense of $80–100 is much less than the cost for 3 full toxicological screens. Aside from marijuana and cocaine, in-office tests are not available for other substances of abuse; however, since the technology of this area is expanding rapidly, it is likely that a full panoply of substances will be available on screening cards in the near future.

An equally important use of such screening tests is for the evaluation of patients with midtrimester cramping and bleeding. Cocaine abuse may lead to uterine contractions and bleeding, presumably because of the vasoconstrictive properties of this drug. The evaluation of bleeding and cramping patients in the second trimester of pregnancy has always been enigmatic, although ultrasound examination can provide useful insights (i.e. placenta previa) in some patients. In many instances, however, no cause is found. Unfortunately, even if substances of abuse are suspected, the time required for quantitative urine toxicology is lengthy and the clinician may need assistance before the results of such examinations are available. The use of rapid screening examinations may be invaluable to obtain this information in a timely fashion. Positive test results can corroborate the clinician's initial impressions and refute the historical data presented by the patient. This information may be used to encourage a patient to seek appropriate psychosocial intervention and to identify a fetus at risk in order to heighten fetal surveillance. It should be stressed that screening examinations are just that; in many instances the clinician may require a full toxicological examination for confirmation of the initial finding.

Antenatal Fetal Surveillance

Fetal well-being should be assessed frequently. This is particularly true during methadone detoxification or the abrupt cessation of cocaine use. Both processes undoubtedly affect the fetus as well as the mother. In the case of rapid methadone detoxification, the sequence of events has been characterized as follows[39]:

- Maternal withdrawal
- Fetal withdrawal
- Fetal hyperactivity
- Intrauterine convulsions
- Passage of meconium
- Strong fetal respiratory movements
- Intrauterine demise or neonatal death

According to Zuspan et al.[39] reduction of methadone dosage by 2 mg/wk obviates this problem.

Similar mechanisms for the abrupt cessation of cocaine use have yet to be clarified. However, since the administration of cocaine may impair fetal oxygenation through catacholamine vasoconstriction of the uteroplacental vessels, it is possible that the degree of fetal hypoxemia is more closely related to prolonged and/or heavy abuse patterns than it is to the abrupt cessation of abuse.

Evidence of fetal hypoxia or stress frequently may be deduced from the presence of meconium in the amniotic fluid of substantial numbers of heroin addicted women. According to Naeye et al.[40] the presence of meconium-laden macrophages, as demonstrated by histologic examination of placentas from heroin-addicted mothers, also suggests that the fetus may be experiencing episodes of hypoxia or other stress, possibly even withdrawal, while in utero. There are no valid means to assess the timing or the extent of the presumed event.

Fetal surveillance should include serial ultrasound assessment of fetal growth and daily fetal movement counts. If the fetus is undergrown, fetal movement is decreased or cocaine is a substance of abuse, weekly biophysical testing should be performed. Biophysical tests include non-stress test, contraction stress test and biophysical profile. In addition, doppler velocity waveform evaluations of uterine and umbilical arteries may be performed in those pregnancies complicated by cocaine abuse or fetal growth retardation.

Post-delivery plans should be formulated prior to delivery. This is particularly true if it is anticipated that the infant may require a longer hospitalization than the mother or if the mother exhibits social or behavioral traits that conceivably would interfere with her parenting role. If infant adoption is contemplated or if sterilization has been requested, appropriate forms, consents, and releases should be available before the anticipated date of delivery.

Labor, Delivery and Post-partum

The management of the pregnant addict's labor frequently is complicated by the fact that her drug habit is unknown to those providing intrapartum care. A high degree of suspicion is required to identify these individuals, as addicted patients often fail to reveal their problem unless a crisis occurs. The presence of needle tracks or abscesses on the skin of a patient in labor with a history of no prenatal care should alert nurses and physicians to possible heroin abuse. Unfortunately, no such stigmata are available to distinguish the cocaine addict or, for that matter, the individual who chronically abuses alcohol or marijuana. In these latter instances labor and delivery personnel may be confronted with an individual exhibiting signs of rhinitis and agitation, early withdrawal or permeating the aroma of marijuana.

Patients actively addicted to heroin commonly remain at home until labor is well advanced, only to arrive at the hospital ready to deliver, often 'high' on a last-minute drug fix taken to alleviate the pain of labor. Self-discharge against medical advice shortly after delivery is a frequent occurrence, often within the first 24 hours.

Should the patient remain longer, friends may help allay her cravings and withdrawal symptoms by providing illicit drugs surrepticiously. Table 2.5 is a summary of the signs and symptoms of maternal opiate withdrawal.

Table 2.5 Signs and symptoms of opiate withdrawal

Early	Late
Craving for drugs	Aching in bones and muscles
Thirst	Regurgitation
Anxiety	Diarrhea
Restlessness	Elevated blood pressure
Lacrimation	Hyperpyrexia
Tremors	Hyperventilation
Hot and cold flashes	Tachycardia
Diaphoresis	Abdominal bloating
Nausea	Cramps
Yawning	Convulsions
Mydriasis	

Table 2.6 Methadone doses in opiate withdrawal*

Signs and symptoms	Initial methadone dose (mg)
Grade I	
Lacrimation, diaphoresis, yawning, restlessness, insomnia	5
Grade II	
Dilated pupils, muscle twitching, myalgia, arthralgia, abdominal pain	10
Grade III	
Tachycardia, hypertension, tachypnea, fever, anorexia, nausea, extreme restlessness	15
Grade IV	
Diarrhea, vomiting, dehydration, hyperglycemia, hypotension, curled-up position	20

*From Fultz and Senay[41]

The drug of choice to stabilize heroin withdrawal in labor is methadone, given intramuscularly. If methadone is given orally, emesis or delayed gastric emptying may interfere with its absorption. Dosage should be based on the severity of the signs and symptoms. Table 2.6 presents guidelines for dose selection, according to Fultz and Senay[41]. The therapeutic effect of intramuscular methadone is not achieved for 30–60 minutes. When with- drawal symptoms are severe, judicious use of a short-acting narcotic may be necessary. Recommended agents include morphine, meperidine (Demerol)[R], methadone, and hydromorphine (Dilaudid)[R]. Pentazocine (Talwin)[R] should *never* be administered, since this analgesic also acts as a potent narcotic antagonist and will precipitate acute withdrawal in an addicted individual[41]. If the patient has been enrolled in a methadone maintenance program, the usual morning dose should be administered, preferably intramuscularly. In most low-dose methadone maintenance programs, a dose of 30 mg/day commonly controls withdrawal symptoms. Once withdrawal symptoms are under control (or if the patient is well maintained and not in withdrawal), the obstetrician is free to use whatever methods of anesthesia or analgesia are deemed necessary to provide pain relief for labor and delivery. In spite of their history of drug abuse and/or methadone maintenance, addicted parturients experience real pain with parturition. Withholding medications in the mistaken belief that these agents contribute to the addictive process is not necessary.

Guidelines for managing labor and the postpartum period are the same as for the non-addicted patient. The infant, however, should be observed closely in the hospital if antepartum maternal drug abuse has been documented. Methadone and cocaine both are excreted in breast milk, and this should be noted when patients request to breastfeed their infants. Blinick et al.[42] measured methadone levels in maternal serum and breast milk; when methadone was present in serum, it was also present in breast milk. The average ratio of methadone concentration in breast milk to that in maternal serum was 0.83. If barbiturates constituted a significant portion of the drugs of abuse, the passively addicted infant should be observed in the hospital for at least 4 to 7 days and possibly longer. Chasnoff et al.[43] have reported neonatal convulsions in a breast feeding infant whose mother was consuming large amounts of cocaine.

The incidence of delivery complications in drug-addicted women compared with non-addicted women may vary somewhat by substance of addiction. The triad of premature rupture of the membranes, preterm delivery, and diminished fetal weight have been long appreciated in women actively addicted to heroin[24] or maintained on methadone[10]. More recently, it has become clear that this triad may also be characteristic for abusers of cocaine[11], combinations of cocaine and opiates[13] and other substances as well.

Cocaine Storm

A disturbing second trimester phenomenon, for the lack of a better term, can be designated as 'Cocaine Storm'. This analogy is appropriate because at the height of a severe storm (rain, snow, sand) a given individual may lose his/her sense of direction and, in selected instances, connection to reality. In cases we recently observed, patients presented themselves to us in the mid-trimester of pregnancy with symptoms of abdominal pain, cramping, and, in some instances, bleeding. These symptoms were accompanied by rather pronounced mental detachment and unconcern. A history of heavy and prolonged cocaine use prior to the onset of symptoms was readily elicited. These women were admitted to the obstetric unit for observation and, once it had been determined that they were not in imminent danger of mid-trimester pregnancy loss, transfer to a chemical dependency unit was advised. Unfortunately, not all patients chose to accept this advice; some left the obstetric unit shortly after their symptoms abated, continued to use cocaine and subsequently lost their pregnancies.

Prolonged cocaine use in the midtrimester of pregnancy is a serious medical and psychosocial emergency. Not only is pregnancy wastage a real possibility, but the mother is at grave risk of a continued deterioration in her reality testing capacity. She is also at risk of death from cerebrovascular, myocardial, or uterine vasoconstrictive events. Whenever possible, such individuals should be offered hospitalization in a psychotherapeutic mileu as soon as her obstetric condition is deemed stable. Upon discharge, psycho-social interventions must continue as an outpatient and the intensity of prenatal contact should be increased, assuming the pregnancy remains viable. Weekly or semi-weekly prenatal visits are reasonable. At these visits the fetal status should be assessed and the mother should receive additional support, advice and counseling from the obstetric care team.

OBSTETRIC AND PERINATAL OUTCOME IN ADDICTED PARTURIENTS: THE NORTHWESTERN EXPERIENCE

This section will summarize pertinent obstetric data from the PCCD by type of addiction. Commentary on opiate addiction were developed following reviews of patients delivered between April 1976 and October 1980[10]. Records of patients with cocaine abuse were reviewed for the years 1983–86[11]. Sonographic data was collected from cocaine-abusing patients delivering between 1983 and 1986[12]. Finally, entire drug-abusing population patients between 1982 and 1986 were reviewed[13].

34

Opiate Addiction: 1976–1980

Demographic Patterns and Patient Profile

Fifty-eight women were delivered of sixty-two infants. Two program participants returned to have a second child, and twin pregnancies occurred in two additional women. The majority (70%) of the patients were under 25 years of age. Caucasian and black patients were roughly equal in numbers. Half the patients had never been married. The remainder were separated or divorced. Of particular interest was the educational background of these women: 41% had completed 12 or more years of formal education.

Antepartum OB History and Risk Factors

Whereas only one-third of the patients were pregnant for the first time, more than half were expecting their first child. One abortion (spontaneous or induced) had been experienced in almost half of the patients. Since these patients were young and abortion had been universally available since 1973, elements of criminality were not part of the history-taking process. Patients averaged almost nine prenatal visits. The various risk factors outlined in the standard Hollister obstetric history were not present in significant numbers. Although intrauterine growth retardation was occasionally suspected because of somewhat small uterine size for dates, subsequent ultrasound observations and delivery data did not confirm these clinical impressions. Smoking was popular (75%); alcohol consumption was not (20%).

Intrapartum and Infant Data

Tables 2.7 and 2.8 list important features of delivery data and immediate neonatal outcome. Spontaneous vaginal delivery occurred in two-thirds of the cases; forceps were used in 20% of patients. Seven patients were delivered by Cesarean section for accepted obstetrical complications. The adjusted percentage of deliveries judged at term by weeks of gestation was greater than 90%. When the weights of all infants were superimposed upon standard profiles for the US, the number of infants below the 50th percentile was slightly more than the number above it, but the difference was not remarkable. With regard to length, infants at term ranked almost equally above and below the 50th percentile. Four term infants were below the 10th percentile for head circumference and five were above the 90th percentile.

Table 2.7 Opiate addiction 1976–80 – obstetric data

	No.	Percentage
Gestational age (weeks)		
30–34	3	5.0
35–37	6	5.0
38–40	45	70.0
41–44	6	10.0
Birthweight (g)		
<1500	1	1.6
1500–1999	1	1.6
2000–2499	11	17.7
2500–2999	24	38.4
3000–3499	12	19.4
>3500	13	21.0

From Rosner et al.[10]

Table 2.8 Opiate addiction 1976–80 – neonatal data

	No.	Percentage
Apgar score at 1 min.		
1–4	4	6.4
5–6	6	9.7
7–9	52	83.8
Apgar score at 5 min.		
5–6	5	4.8
7–10	59	95.2
Medical complications:		
Respiratory distress syndrome	1	1.6
Meconium aspiration	1	1.6
Sepsis, culture negative	4	6.9
Other (jaundice)	5	8.1
None	51	82.2

From Rosner et al.[10]

Infants of drug-addicted mothers had a slight trend toward lower weights at term, and this trend was also observed in length and head circumference measurements. Table 2.9 compares average infant weights in our program with other recently published data from similar patients. Of comparative interest, the average weight of infants delivered at the Cook County Hospital between 1969 and 1972 to mothers actively addicted to heroin was 2393 g, and the percentage of infants whose weights were less than 2500 g was 52%[25].

Table 2.9 Mean weights of infants delivered of mothers in methadone programs, 1976–1982 – publications

Author	Year of publication	Mean weight (g)
Rosner et al.	1982	2935
Stimmel and Adamsons*	1976	2933
Kendall et al.**	1976	2961
Newman et al.***	1976	2738 [+]

[+] Mothers receiving 40 mg/d had infants with a mean of 2806 g

* Stimmel, B. and Adamsons, K. (1976). Narcotic dependency in pregnancy: methadone maintenance compared to use of street drugs. *J. Am. Med. Assoc.*, **235**, 1121

** Kendall, S.R., Albin, S., Lowinson, J., Berle, B., Eidelman, A.J. and Garner, L.M. (1976). Differential effects of maternal heroin and methadone use on birthweight. *Pediatrics*, **58**, 681

*** Newman, R.G., Bashkow, S. and Calko, D. (1975). Results of 313 consecutive live births of infants delivered to patients in the New York City methadone maintenance treatment program. *Am. J. Obstet. Gynecol.*, **121**, 233

Cocaine Addiction: 1983–86

Demographic Patterns and Patient Profile

Seventy patients whose primary drug of abuse was cocaine were studied along with an equal number of controls matched for age, parity, socio-economic class, tobacco use and medical complications. Cocaine addicts had significantly more abortions (not differentiated between spontaneous and elective) compared to controls (1.7 ± 1.5 vs. 0.7 ± 1.2, respectively). The mean number of prenatal visits was significantly less in the cocaine patients.

Obstetric Data

Table 2.10 summarizes the differences between cocaine-abusing patients and controls for gestational age at delivery and birthweight. The incidence of preterm labor (prior to 37 weeks' gestation) was significantly greater in cocaine abusing patients than controls (21.4% vs. 1.4%). The difference in preterm delivery rates was equally apparent (24.3% vs. 2.9%, respectively). In addition, the proportion of pregnancies complicated by abruptio placentae and congenital anomalies were greater in cocaine-abusing pregnancies compared to controls (7.1% and 5.7% vs. 1.4% and 1.4%, respectively). The small number of patients prevented these differences from reaching statistical significance; however, clinically these differences are alarming.

Table 2.10 Cocaine addiction 1983–1986 – obstetric data

	Cocaine patients (n = 70)	Controls (n = 70)	Significance (p value)
Preterm labor*	15 (21.4%)	1 (1.4%)	<.001
Preterm delivery*	17 (24.3%)	2 (2.9%)	<.0005
Gestational age at delivery	37.1 ± 3.6	39.3 ± 2.0	<.0001
Birthweight	2853 ± 698	3382 ± 551	<.00001
Low birthweight +	16 (22.9%)	3 (4.3%)	<.005
SGA**	13 (18.6%)	2 (2.9%)	<.0001

*   Prior to 37 weeks' gestation
** Birthweight <10th percentile by Brenners birth weight curve
+   Birthweight <2500 grams

Adapted from MacGregor et al.[11]

Neonatal Data

Low Apgar scores at one and five minutes, low umbilical artery pH values and the proportion of pregnancies complicated by meconium staining or abnormal fetal heart rate tracings were similar for infants of cocaine-abusing mothers and controls.

The study group was divided into two subgroups: those who abused only cocaine (n = 24) and those who abused cocaine plus any one of the following: opiates, marijuana, barbituates, amphetamines, phencyclidine, benzodiaze-pines or LSD (n = 46). Although the differences between these subsets were not statistically different, several interesting trends were clearly apparent. The mean birthweight of infants whose mothers abused only cocaine was 2677 g compared to 2944 g for those who abused cocaine and other substances as well. Low (<2500 g) birthweight was twice as common (33% vs. 17%) among mothers whose sole drug of abuse was cocaine compared to those who abused cocaine and other drugs. Of interest was the fact that infants whose birthweights were less than the tenth percentile of standard birthweight curves[44] were three times more common in the mothers whose only drug of abuse was cocaine compared to cocaine plus other substances (25% vs. 8.7% respectively). Of additional interest is the fact that the mean infant weight for babies born to 'pure' cocaine abusing mothers was lower than the average weights commonly reported from methadone programs between the years 1976 and 1982 (Table 2.9). While it is clear that these diverse populations are not comparable for many reasons, this low birth-weight is alarming. It approaches the average weight of 2393 g reported by Clark et al.[24] among 104 drug-addicted (primarily heroin) patients delivered between 1969 and 1972 at the Cook County Hospital in Chicago.

Ultrasonic data was evaluated for forty-three of the mothers who were addicted to cocaine[12]. Suboptimal fetal growth was noted in approximately 46% of study patients. In particular, 17 (39.5%) fetuses exhibited a significant diminution in abdominal circumference, and 3 showed diminution of both head and body perimeters. Moreover, biparietal diameter measurements obtained in the third trimester fell significantly below those expected in normal fetuses, whereas head circumference values remained within normal limits, suggesting late-onset dolichocephaly.

MANAGEMENT OF THE ADDICTION/PREGNANCY COMPLEX

Opiate Addiction

Dole and Nyswander[45] first utilized methadone in 1965 for the clinical management of heroin addicts. Clinical trials of methadone use in pregnant women were reported in 1969[46]. The early initial enthusiasm for methadone substitution was followed by a serious re-examination of the merits and drawbacks of using this medication in pregnancy.

The six potential approaches to the management of the pregnant opiate addict follow:

(1)   prenatal care and support with no attempt to alter the addiction pattern;
(2)   acute detoxification;

(3)   slow detoxification with methadone;
(4)   methadone maintenance;
(5)   low dose methadone maintenance combined with psychosocial counseling;
(6)   drug-free communities.

Supporting the patient prenatally without altering her addiction pattern implies continued procurement of 'street' drugs and cyclic episodes of the 'highs' and 'lows' followed by withdrawal symptoms and occasional drug craving. Such behavior predictably is associated with higher risks of maternal and fetal complications.

When a pregnant woman undergoes acute withdrawal or detoxification ('cold turkey'), the fetus also experiences withdrawal. However, the fetus is less able to tolerate the insults of withdrawal than its mother, and intrauterine death may result. Elective acute withdrawal or detoxification during pregnancy is almost never advised. Zuspan *et al.*[39] measured amino acid levels in amniotic fluid of addicted prenatal patients and found that significant increases in epinephrine and norepinephrine levels occurred in response to relatively mild reductions in methadone dosages. These investigators interpreted their findings as evidence of fetal distress and strongly recommended detoxification not be attempted during pregnancy.

Our own experience is somewhat more encouraging. Depending on the initial dosage, small reductions have been made on a weekly or bi-weekly basis in selected patients. Maternal and fetal assessments were made routinely. Since 1975 we have reduced the dosage of methadone in 15 women during pregnancy without serious maternal or fetal side effects. Some prenatal clinics advocate slow detoxification with methadone and subsequent complete withdrawal. However, this method of treatment may fail unless the social and psychological aspects of addiction are considered concomitantly.

High doses (80 mg or more/day) of methadone can be used to effect a 'blockade'. The rationale for this therapy is that tolerance develops at high dosages and the addict is unlikely to get her usual 'high' if illicit heroin is also used. While this perception may be true, the patient who presents in pregnancy using 100 mg of methadone or more on a daily basis represents a true treatment dilema. If kept at that dose, the newborn is likely to experience prolonged withdrawal and difficulty in adjusting after birth. Even if the dose is reduced, neonatal problems may be diminished but not obviated. These circumstances notwithstanding, the patient's ability to function at these high doses may be impaired to such a degree that the parenting process becomes a problem. In contrast, low-dose methadone maintenance programs work on the premise that all opiates exert an adverse effect on the fetus. Accordingly, the pregnant addict is maintained on the lowest dose possible (5–40 mg/day).

In drug-free communities, patients are offered drug withdrawal, detoxification, and abstinence. Unless the addict is drug-free upon entry into the program, acute detoxification usually is mandated. This approach is often successful in the general population of drug addicts. However, in the pregnant addict, acute detoxification and withdrawal is discouraged for the reasons discussed above.

The Medical Use of Methadone

Since the pharmacologic actions of methadone are similar to those of heroin, the abuse potential is comparable. However, the maternal effects of methadone use may be different from those of heroin because methadone can be obtained legally and often is supplied without charge. Although maintenance on the lowest possible dose is optimal, this dose must be sufficient to discourage supplementation with illicitly obtained heroin or methadone. If the maintenance dosage is too low, abuse with other drugs, including tranquilizers, sedatives or alcohol often helps alleviate withdrawal symptoms.

The initial dose of methadone must be calculated with caution. Ideally, this dose should be based on a combination of physical examination and signs and symptoms of opiate withdrawal. The regimen described by Fultz and Senay[41] is shown in Table 2.6.

Merits and Disadvantages of Methadone Use

At one time methadone was considered a panacea. Unlike heroin, which is short-acting and pharmacologically available for only about 4 hours, methadone's activity spans approximately 24 hours. The therapeutic rationale for methadone use is to sustain the addict and hold withdrawal symptoms in abeyance.

In pregnancy, the avoidance of the cyclic craving and withdrawal is especially important to the fetus. Methadone helps to establish a stabilized drug milieu for the fetus; theoretically, this stability should improve neonatal outcome. Critical evaluation of clinical experience with methadone in pregnancy indicates that maternal complications are decreased and fetal outcome is improved[7], probably due to the mother having had prenatal care. Unfortunately, the infants of mothers who have used methadone are not immune from problems. The merits of methadone use are generally confined to the prenatal period and the disadvantages to the neonatal period, (Table

41

2.11). Many disadvantages are associated with high-dose (80–120 mg daily) methadone maintenance and are eliminated by low-dose methadone maintenance (<40 mg).

Table 2.11 Observations on methadone use in pregnancy

Advantages:
- Decreased incidence of low birthweight infants
- Decreased incidence of prematurity
- Decreased incidence of obstetric complications
- Increased organ size and total cell number as compared with those of infants of untreated heroin-addicted mothers

Disadvantages:
- Increased incidence of low Apgar scores
- Greater neonatal weight loss
- Increased frequency, severity, and length of withdrawal symptoms as compared with those infants of untreated heroin-addicted mothers
- Increased incidence of convulsive seizures
- Increased newborn serum bilirubin levels as compared with those of infants of untreated heroin-addicted mothers
- Decreased visual orientation and following response in the infant
- Initially depressed suck rates
- Longer hospitalization and treatment of neonatal withdrawal symptoms

Most participants in methadone maintenance programs do not use this drug exclusively. The problem of 'chipping' with heroin or other drugs thus adds a variable which is impossible to evaluate or control. Programs that routinely screen urines report that as many as 80% of their pregnant patients test positive at least once; a large percentage of them submit 'dirty' urine specimens on multiple occasions. In spite of these problems, properly supervised methadone maintenance appears to exert a positive effect on pregnancy outcome. Serious questions have been raised, however, concerning the neonatal as well as the long-term effects of methadone on infant development. In any such evaluations, not only is the extent and duration of intrauterine drug exposure important, but the effects of postnatal environment and the mother–child interaction must also be considered.

Cocaine Addiction

Comparitively little data exists regarding therapy of cocaine addiction in pregnant women. Among the reasons for this are first, the recent rapid escalation in the numbers of individuals using cocaine (i.e. since 1980); and second, the learning period required to appreciate the inherent differences between addiction to cocaine compared to opiates. It is much more difficult to achieve abstinence and a salutory pregnancy outcome in a cocaine addict than it is to maintain a pregnant woman on methadone or substitute this agent for heroin. Not only is methadone a replacement for heroin from a psychological point of view, but it alleviates symptoms of physical withdrawal from heroin. To date, no substitute has been found for cocaine that provides a similar feeling or prevents withdrawal. As a result, the clinician has little to offer his patients except exhortations, good advice and psychosocial intervention (not necessarily in that order). Whether these activities will be effective in reducing the frequency and quantity of cocaine use depends on many factors, most of which are beyond the control of the individual clinician and/or drug program. In the largest series published to date regarding obstetric outcomes in pregnant cocaine addicts, MacGregor *et al.*[11] noted that only 1/3 of their patients were able to maintain a drug-free state after enrollment for prenatal care. Outcome differences among the addicts who remained drug free compared to those who did not were not measured in this report.

Hospitalization in a chemical dependence program of a psychiatric facility is often appropriate for pregnant cocaine addicts, but this alternative is expensive and/or not always acceptable to the patient. Forcible committment is an unlikely possibility unless the patient is frankly psychotic. The advantages of voluntary hospitalization are several and include: (1) severing ties with drug-abusing companions; (2) removal from a stressful environment; (3) reintroduction of normal sleeping and eating patterns; (4) initiation of psychotherapeutic rehabilitation and (5) treatment of underlying medical problems.

Failure to control cocaine abuse in pregnancy may preceed an obstetric disaster. The loss of control observed in patients after prolonged cocaine use may obliterate any internal awareness that their drug-seeking behavior adversely affects the pregnancy by greatly increasing the risk of infant and/or maternal complications. Moreover, if pregnancy terminates preterm and with adverse outcome to the fetus, the mother may become severely depressed by guilt and regret for the manner in which the pregnancy terminated.

The concern of the general obstetrician for the pregnant cocaine abuser should include the following: (1) an ability to recognize the patient in whom cocaine use may preceed serious pregnancy complications; and (2) the capacity to refer such patients to appropriate facilities for specialized obstetric care and/or prolonged psychosocial intervention when deemed appropriate.

SUMMARY

Much work remains to be done in the field of drug addiction and pregnancy. Among the most urgent needs are the following:

(1)   determine the true incidence of substance abuse among pregnant women;

(2)   develop more efficient and less costly methods of screening for a variety of substances which have the potential for abuse during pregnancy;

(3)   determine which medical and/or psychosocial intervention strategies are most beneficial for specific addictions;

(4)   determine the extent to which the addictive process or addictive processes contribute to neonatal and maternal morbidity and mortality;

(5)   determine how to prevent long-term developmental sequelae in the children of addicted mothers;

(6)   determine how to curtail the transgenerational hold of the addictive aspects of the maternal personality on the next generation.

REFERENCES

1.   de Quincey, T. (1822). *Confessions of an Opium Eater*
2.   Danis, R.P., Newton, M. and Keith, L.G. (1981). Pregnancy and alcohol. *Current Problems in Obstetrics and Gynecology*, IV (Chicago: Year Book Medical Publishers)
3.   Lemoine, P., Haronsseau, H. and Borteyru, J.P. (1968). Les enfants de parents alcoholiques. *Ouest Med.*, 25, 477
4.   Jones, K.L., Smith, D.W. and Ulleland, C.N. (1973). Patterns of malformation in offspring of alcoholic mothers. *Lancet*, 1, 1267
5.   Jones, K.L. and Smith, D.W. (1978). Recognition of fetal alcohol syndrome. *N. Engl. J. Med.*, 298, 1063
6.   Heinonen, O.P., Sloane, D. and Shapiro, S. (1977). *Birth Defects and Drugs in Pregnancy.* (Littleton, Mass.: Publishing Sciences Group)
7.   Beeley, L. (1986). Adverse effects of drugs in later pregnancy. *Clin. Obstet. Gynecol.*, 13, 197–214
8.   Eriksson, M., Larson, G. and Zetterstrom, R. (1981). Amphetamine addiction and pregnancy II. Pregnancy, delivery and neonatal period socio-economic aspects. *Acta Obstet. Gynecol. Scand.*, 60, 253–9
9.   Smith, C.G. and Ash, R.H. (1987). Drug abuse and reproduction. *Fertil. Steril.*, 48, 355–73
10. Rosner, M.A., Keith, L. and Chasnoff, I. (1982). The Northwestern University drug dependence program: the impact of intensive prenatal care on labor and delivery outcomes. *Am. J. Obstet. Gynecol.*, 144, 23–27
11. MacGregor, S.N., Keith, L.G., Chasnoff, I.J., Rosner, M.A., Chisum, G.M., Shaw, P. and Minogue, J.P. (1987). Cocaine use during pregnancy: adverse perinatal outcome. *Am. J. Obstet. Gynecol.*, 157, 686–690

12. Mitchell, M., Sabbagha, R., Keith, L., MacGregor, S., Mota, J. and Minoque, J. (1988). Ultrasonic growth parameter in fetuses of mothers with primary addiction to cocaine. *Am. J. Obstet. Gynecol.* (In press)
13. Keith, L.G., MacGregor, S.N., Friedell, S. and Chasnoff, I.J. (1988). Substance abuse in pregnant women: recent experience at the Perinatal Center for Chemical Dependence of Northwestern Memorial Hospital, (submitted for publication)
14. Ward, S.L., Schutz, S. and Kirshna, V. (1986). Abnormal sleeping ventilatory patterns in infants of substance-abusing mothers. *Am. J. Dis. Child.*, **140**, 1015 – 20
15. Chasnoff, I.J., Burns, W.J., Schnoll, S. and Burns, K.A. (1985). Cocaine use in pregnancy. *N. Engl. J. Med.*, **313**, 666 – 9
16. Chasnoff, I. (1986). Alcohol use in pregnancy. In Chasnoff, I.J. (ed.) *Drug Use in Pregnancy: Mother and Child*, pp. 75 – 78. (Lancaster: MTP Press)
17. Wilsnack, S.C., Klasseu, A.D. and Wilsnack, R.W. (1981). Drinking and reproductive dysfunction among women in a 1981 national survey. *Alcoholism*, **8**, 451 – 8
18. Hallstedt, C., Dahlgren, L. and Rydberg, V. (1983). Outcome of pregnancy in women treated in an alcohol clinic. *Acta Psychiatr. Scand.*, **67**, 236 – 48
19. Hallstedt, C., Dahlgren, L. and Rydberg, V. (1983). Alcoholic women in fertile age treated in an alcohol clinic. *Acta Psychiatr. Scand.*, **67**, 195 – 204
20. Kyllerman, M., Aronson, M., Sabel, K.G. *et al.* (1985). The children of alcoholic mothers. Growth and motor performance compared to matched controls. *Acta Paediatr. Scand.*, **74**, 20 – 6
21. Aronson, M., Kyllerman, M., Sabel, K.G. *et al.* (1985). Children of alcoholic mothers: developmental, perceptual and behavioral characteristics as compared to matched controls. *Acta Paediatr. Scand.*, **74**, 27 – 35
22. Schnoll, S. (1986). Pharmacologic basis of perinatal addiction. In Chasnoff, I.J. (ed.) *Drug Use in Pregnancy: Mother and Child*, pp. 7 – 16 (Lancaster: MTP Press)
23. Keith, L., Donald, W., Rosner, M., Mitchell, M. and Bianchi, J. (1986). Obstetric aspects of perinatal addiction. In Chasnoff, I.J. (ed.) *Drug Use in Pregnancy: Mother and Child*, pp. 23 – 41. (Lancaster: MTP Press)
24. Clark, D., Keith, L., Pildes, R. *et al.* (1974). Drug dependent obstetric patients. *J. Obstet. Gynecol. Nurs.*, **3**, 17 – 20
25. Vargas, G.C., Pildes, R.S., Vidyasager, D. *et al.* (1975). Effects of maternal heroin addiction on 67 liveborn neonates: withdrawal symptoms, small body size and small head circumference. *Clin. Pediatr.*, **14**, 751 – 7
26. Finnegan, L.P. (ed.) (1978). *Drug Dependence in Pregnancy: Clinical Management of Mother and Child*. National Institute of Drug Abuse, Service Research Monograph Series. (Rockville MD:U.S. Government Printing Office)
27. Fishburne, P.M., Abelson, H.I. and Cisin, I. (1983). *National Household Survey on Drug Abuse: National Institute of Drug and Alcohol Abuse Capsules 1982*. (Rockville MD: Dept. Health and Human Services)
28. Chambers, C.D. and Griffey, M.S. (1975). Use of legal substance within the general population: the sex and age variables. *Addict. Dis.*, **2**, 7 – 15
29. Viner, R. (1988). Opiate addiction, pregnancy and mothering. *Thesis dissertation*, Northwestern University
30. Bowen, M. (1972). Towards the differentiation of a self in one's own family. In Framo, J.L. (ed.) *Family Interactions*. (New York: Springer-Verlag)
31. Bowen, M. (1978). *Family Therapy in Clinical Practice*. (New York: Jason Aronson)
32. Goulden, E.C., Littlefield, D.C., Putoff, O.E. and Sievert, A.C. (1964). Menstrual abnormalities associated with heroin addiction. *Am. J. Obstet. Gynecol.*, **90**, 155 – 8
33. Santen, R.J., Sofsky, J., Bilie, N. *et al.* (1975). Mechanism of action of narcotics in the production of menstrual dysfunction in women. *Fertil. Steril.*, **26**, 538 – 45
34. Rementaria, J., Janakammal, S. and Hollander, M. (1975). Multiple births in drug addicted women. *Am. J. Obstet. Gynecol.*, **122**, 958 – 60
35. Abrams, C.A. (1982). Cytogenetic risks to the offspring of pregnant addicts. *Addict. Dis.*, **2**, 63 – 77

36. Sabaggha, R.E., Hughey, M. and Depp, R. (1986). Growth adjusted sonographic age: a simplified method. *Obstet. Gynecol.*, **51**, 383 – 6
37. Zuspan, F.P. and Rayburn, W.F. (1986). Drug abuse during pregnancy. In Rayburn, W.F. and Zuspan, F.P. (eds.) *Drug Therapy in Obstetrics and Gynecology.* (Norwalk, CN: Appleton-Century-Crofts)
38. Keith, L.G., Sciarra, J.C., MacGregor, S.N. and Sciarra, J.S. (1988). Routine screening for cocaine and marijuana in urine of pregnant women. (Unpublished data)
39. Zuspan, F., Gumpel, J., Mejia-Zelaya, A. *et al.* (1975). Fetal stress from methadone withdrawal. *Am. J. Obstet. Gynecol.*, **122**, 43 – 8
40. Naeye, R., Blane, W., Leblanc, W. *et al.* (1973). Fetal complications of maternal heroin addiction: abnormal growth, infections and episodes of stress. *J. Pediatr.*, **83**, 1055 – 8
41. Fultz, J. and Senay, E. (1975). Guidelines for the management of hospitalized narcotic addicts. *Ann. Intern. Med.*, **82**, 815 – 8
42. Blinick, G., Inturrisi, C., Jerez, E. *et al.* (1975). Methadone assays in pregnant women and progeny. *Am. J. Obstet. Gynecol.*, **121**, 617 – 19
43. Chasnoff, I.J., Lewis, D.E. and Squires, L. (1987). Cocaine intoxication in a breastfed infant. *Pediatrics*, **80**, 836 – 8
44. Brenner, W.E., Edelman, D.A. and Hendricks, C.H. (1976). A standard of fetal growth for the United States of America. *Am. J. Obstet. Gynecol.*, **126**, 555-7
45. Dole, V.P. and Nyswander, M.E. (1965). A medical treatment for diacetylmorphine (heroin) addiction: a clinical trial with methadone hydrochloride. *J. Am. Med. Assoc.*, **193**, 646 – 50
46. Wallach, R.C., Jerez, E. and Blinick, G. (1969). Pregnancy and menstrual function in narcotic addicts treated with methadone: the methadone maintenance program. *Am. J. Obstet. Gynecol.*, **105**, 1226 – 30

This chapter substantially reproduces material to be published in *Gynecology and Obstetrics*, Vol.3, Chapter 31, J.B. Lippincott Company, Philadelphia, 1989, with permission of the editor.

3

A Treatment Model of Nursing Care for Pregnant Chemical Abusers

Bonnie Michaels, Melinda Noonan, Sandy Hoffman and Rita Allen Brennan

In 1968 a special committee on alcoholism and narcotics conducting a survey on female opiate addiction estimated that there were 110,000 heroin addicts in the United States. In 1971, just 3 years later, a special study of the House of Representatives placed the figure at 250,000[1]. In 1973, the National Institute of Drug Abuse estimated that 415,200 addicts were concentrated in 24 metropolitan areas, an increase of almost four-fold in only five years[2]. Although these studies did not provide statistics on the number of female addicts included, the estimates have ranged between 20 and 30%.

It is thus astonishing that so little attention has been paid to pregnant addicts. Nor, until recently, has anyone studied addicts with children or neonatal addiction. We do know that the number of female addicts is increasing dramatically[3]. In 1976, in New York City, the Addiction Services Agency reported that 80% of female addicts were between 15 and 35[4]. Thus, the majority of female addicts are of childbearing age.

Due to the unwillingness of females to be identified as addicts and their fear of reprisals from the courts, it is probable that many pregnant addicts escape detection. A significant number also may self deliver without a physician in attendance. Thus pregnancies of addicts, which until the late 1970s were not even studied, still have been underestimated. Estimates of neonatal mortality have ranged from 7 to 20% due to unreported stillborns or deaths from neonatal withdrawal[5].

Cusky, Berger and Densen-Berger, in a paper on issues in the treatment of female addiction, examined the barriers to recruiting female addicts and ways in which they are discouraged from treatment programs[5].

One problem is that most substance abuse programs restrict treatment of pregnant women and mothers. Centers that do offer treatment rarely have day care facilities or programs for children. Intimidated mothers fear they may have to give up their children to relatives or the courts if they identify themselves as chemically dependent, so they avoid treatment.

Also, many programs require that every addicted family member with whom the addict lives enter treatment. Because of the dominant male addicts and excessive dependency among female addicts, many of these addicts seek no treatment at all. The majority of treatment programs are mixed sex programs where women might be less likely to enroll.

The literature devoted to female addicts has been sparse, compared to that dealing with men. Because a treatment model for female addiction has not been developed, most programs operate from the perspective of male oriented treatment models; these are inappropriate to the needs of female patients and probably discourage a significant proportion of women from entering treatment. Female addicts, many of whom lack assertiveness and who may have lower self-esteem than their male counterparts, also may be disinclined to enter treatment centers that often provide a strict regime of punishment and confrontation. Many women feel extremely vulnerable to tearing down sessions, especially when males are present.

In a study by Colten in 1977, female addicts were found to be more disposed to severe depression and have a poorer self-concept. Addicted women feel a greater degree of victimization[6]. In programs where pregnant addicts are admitted, additional difficulties arise pertaining to medical and obstetrical problems seen during the pregnancy. We also know that chemical abuse affects the health of the newborn. The ideal program for pregnant chemically-dependent women must address the medical, obstetrical, psychological and neonatal/pediatric needs of the woman and her baby.

The importance of attending to the emotional needs of the pregnant woman is underscored by the finding that groups that receive psychosocial support have higher treatment retention records and lower incidence of problems than those who do not receive such support[7].

A new approach to counseling pregnant chemically-dependent women is emerging, building upon new theories about the biological, psychological and cultural characteristics of women. This is a new client population whose non-traditional needs and goals demand the development of alternative intervention strategies.

As a result, a common nursing framework applicable to these high-risk women and their special needs which is coordinated and integrated with medical care services provides for the availability of comprehensive patient education programs.

Maximizing opportunities for discussion and education is the key, we feel, to high client compliance. This dissemination of education and coordination of care using a multidisciplinary format is a major foundation in the delivery of nursing care to this target population. Providing confidence in parenting skills leads to self-esteem, and enables the nurse to continue to assess and implement interventive measures and follow-up, meeting client needs across a continuum.

DEVELOPING PARENTING SKILLS

In the history of adult development, parents have come to accept the myth that babies cry, parents please, and babies stop crying. Few parents understand that at times babies cry and cannot be appeased. Instead some parents assume they are inadequate parents.

Parenting classes should assist parents in overcoming these harmful conclusions by teaching parents realistic expectations of themselves. At Northwestern Memorial Hospital a series of five classes is offered to new parents six times a year. Each class session is two hours long. An afternoon class is offered for mothers and their infants and an evening class is offered for couples and their babies. The focus of discussion and lecture each week is different.

The first week is an introductory session with parents sharing their prenatal, labor and delivery, and postpartum experiences. Baby care is the focus of the second class with special attention given to infant growth and development, child safety, accident prevention, coping with a sick baby, and infant nutrition. Parents choose, by the assessment tools described later in this account and by their questions, the areas in which they are most interested. By the third week, parents have become comfortable enough with one another to begin discussing feelings about the many changes in their lives since they have become parents. Since parents are encouraged in this class to regain some of the pleasurable activities of their lives before the baby's birth, it becomes important to discuss the issues of returning to work, baby sitters, and travelling with the baby.

The fourth class is devoted entirely to marital relationships, especially partner communications. By the fifth class, parents are ready to look to future areas of their child's development and to weigh the pros and cons of having another child. Child spacing becomes a topic of great concern.

To establish each parent's particular interests and current concerns, two forms are completed during the first class session. The first form lists fourteen separate items and the parents indicate their interest in these topics. On the parents interest forms, the parents rank in descending order of importance: stages of infant development, play and stimulation, coping with a sick baby, safety and common accidents, local programs and resources, nursing, feeding, and nutrition, leaving child with a babysitter, how normal is child's behavior and development, handling baby's crying, adjusting to parenthood, changes in husband–wife relationship, schedules, spouse–baby relationship and baby equipment.

On the current concerns form parents are asked to list any specific concerns they have or any topics they want specifically addressed during the course. When compiling the data, the parent's requests are arranged into the categories listed on the parents interest form. Once again, parent's concerns are listed in descending order of importance: nursing, feeding, and nutrition, schedules, leaving child with baby sitter, handling baby's crying, stages of infant development, play and stimulation, adjusting to parenthood, safety and common accidents, coping with a sick baby, local programs and resources, changes in husband/wife relationship and baby equipment.

There were some discrepancies with the ranking of importance on the parent's interest forms and the specific questions and information requests listed on the current concerns form. The notable differences were:

	Parents' interest	*Current concerns*
Stages of infant development	1	5
Play and stimulation	2	6
Coping with a sick baby	3	9
Safety and common accidents	4	8
Nursing, feeding and nutrition	6	1
Handling baby's crying	9	4
Adjusting to parenthood	10	7
Schedules	12	2

Surprisingly enough, changes in husband/wife relationship ranked the same on both forms, number 11 of 14 items. However, during the class period and on the course evaluation tool, this is an item most parents are eager to discuss. Parents turn to one another for reassurance that the changes in their marital relationship are not unique. Class sizes must remain small (a maximum of seven couples or ten mothers) to allow for these comparisons.

The physical environment for parenting classes must be different from the traditional classroom setting. The ideal arrangement would be a living room type atmosphere. Arm chairs are a very important consideration. More often than not infants need to be fed during the class period, and it is very uncomfortable to do this without arm support. Two tables are set up as changing tables at either side of the room. The remaining tables are placed together in the middle of the room to form a large rectangle so when parents are seated around the tables they will be facing one another. Ample space is provided between chairs to allow parents to have their baby's stroller next to them. Likewise, the table surface area is large enough to allow parents to place their infants on blankets or in infant seats in front of them. Plenty of hot water must be available to parents to warm baby's bottle or to cleanse dropped pacifiers. Restroom facilities need to be nearby since there are no official break times during the class period. Refreshments of coffee, tea, ice water and juice are arranged in a self-serve fashion in the room.

The ambiance of the room must be warm, comfortable, and inviting. Parents should be invited to move around freely during the class period so they can help themselves to refreshments, change a diaper, fix a bottle, or 'soothe a fussy baby'. In the first class session and in all subsequent sessions, as needed, the instructor must reassure parents that infant crying is to be expected and should be accepted as a normal course of events. It is also helpful if the instructor volunteers to hold and soothe a fussy baby since it is a wonderful way to role model for the parents. Mothers also need to be reassured that breastfeeding will be accepted and indeed welcomed whenever necessary and wherever they are comfortable. Breastfeeding mothers are encouraged to remain with the group instead of going off into a corner.

A variety of teaching strategies must be employed when working with parents in such a distracting environment. No one strategy will work consistently, and flexibility is the key to success. If every baby in class is crying, parents will not be able to hear lecture material or view a film; thus turning this situation into a discussion and role-modeling opportunity is often the best approach. Questions such as, 'What are the most helpful techniques you've learned to soothe a crying baby?' or 'Did you know before you had a baby, that babies cry as much as they do?' are good openers for a discussion on handling baby's crying, even if that was not the proposed topic for discussion at that class.

In the 'Beyond the Birth Experience' classes, films, videos, concisely written handouts, thought-provoking exercises, discussions and lectures are all used interchangeably. There are no topics that cannot be adapted to each of the modes mentioned. Generally, however, the first class is mainly discussion, the second mainly lecture. The third, fourth and fifth classes are a combination of films, exercises, lecture and discussion. Questions are encouraged throughout whether they pertain to the topic at hand or not. The importance of maintaining an open, non-judgemental atmosphere cannot be overemphasized.

Handouts are extremely important for all baby-care topics since parents are not usually in a position to take notes and need the reassurance that the material discussed will be available to them, as needed, in the future. A reading list is also helpful to refer parents to a more indepth understanding of a particular topic.

There are three written exercises utilized in the course. The first exercise is called 'What's Wrong With This Picture?'. Parents are given a drawing in which nineteen unsafe situations can be discerned (i.e. smoldering cigarette next to unattended infant). Most parents are asked to think back to the time before they knew they would become parents, specifically concentrating on how they spent their time in an average week. The participants are then given a blank sheet of paper and pencil and asked to draw a large circle. They are then further instructed to divide the circle into segments as they would a pie, determining the size of the pie piece by the amount of time they spent at the activity they have assigned to the piece. After this pie is completed the parents are asked to now turn the paper over and do the same thing thinking of how they spent their time now. The discussion about adjustments to parenting begins by parents comparing their two pies.

The third exercise is a two-page questionnaire given to each mother and each father called 'Who Does What?'. The mothers and fathers are instructed to complete these questionnaires separately with no discussion until they have each completed the assignment. The form lists household and baby-care tasks with a scale of how often each spouse completes each task. Another scale is for spouses to indicate whether they feel the other spouse should take more or less responsibility for each task. After the forms are completed the mates exchange forms and discuss discrepencies. This exercise leads very naturally into a discussion of couple communication.

Further discussion of marital relationships and the adjustments to parenthood are stimulated by the use of the film *First Child, Second Thoughts*. The film provides a glimpse into the lives of five couples as they discuss the changes in their lives since the birth of their first child. The film broadens the scope of discussion by adding five more sets of experiences for parents in the class to relate to.

As indicated by the parents interests forms and the current concerns forms, parents desire information regarding infant development. *Journey Through The First Year of Life* is a videotape which gives parents that information in a concise, easily understandable format. Dr Burton White is the host of the videotape distributed by *The American Baby*. Infant development is demonstrated in a sequential manner with many helpful suggestions for parent – infant interaction. These demonstrations of infant stimulation are uncomplicated and easy to implement. Most parents today are overwhelmed by the marketing of educational toys and programs. This film repeatedly points out that these elaborate and expensive toys are unnecessary.

The film is divided into several segments so that it can be shown at several different sessions. The segments demonstrating the first three months can be used during the first class after discussion about the early postpartum days. The baby-care class can be augmented with the three to six month segment of the videotape. When feasible, the last segments of the videotape covering seven months to twelve months are useful for the planning hopefully inspired in the last class.

The one mistake that must be avoided with all parenting classes is that of becoming so involved in formalized teaching strategies that the most obvious strategy is ignored: parents role modeling for one another. The role of the group facilitator is to continually focus on the positive parenting skills demonstrated by the participants. Questions asked by participants during class sessions can often be answered by other parents if they are allowed to do so. Since chemically dependent parents, in particular, often lack proper role models in their lives, the need to point out positive role models among other class members is especially important for them.

Our society supports the belief that mothering and, to a lesser extent, fathering, are innate abilities. 'Troubled' parents need support and education, not 'good' parents. This belief of our society is crippling the family support movement. Agencies, private benefactors, researchers, and many others have proven time and again that with the proper education and support, the overwhelming majority of parents can raise happy, healthy, productive members of society. Health professionals are in the ideal position to tip the scales in favor of families. Parents need to know that perinatal education does not end with the baby bath demonstration on the postpartum unit. With the help of all concerned health professionals, parenting classes can become as accepted and as available as Lamaze Classes.

PARENTING THE PREMATURE INFANT

Various authors[8-12] have described the birth of a normal full-term infant as a crisis for most parents. When there is a premature baby this crisis is heightened. Parenting a premature infant is difficult under the best of circumstances. When a parent is chemically dependent, effective parenting becomes even more difficult.

A premature birth brings with it a conflict between expectation and reality. Most parents expect a 'Gerber baby'. A premature infant is hardly a 'Gerber baby'. It is often small, frail, weak and even ugly. Parents are left to mesh their ideal image with the reality of their premature infant.

A premature birth causes many emotional reactions in parents. Stress, anxiety, guilt, anger, fear and failure are frequently cited responses[13-16]. Anxiety and guilt may be intensified when the chemically dependent parent feels responsible for the baby's early birth. Some mothers will indeed make the association between drug abuse and prematurity, while most will not. It is important that nurses educate parents about the effects of drug abuse, to provide honest answers to their questions, while being supportive of them as parents.

53

Caplan, Mason and Kaplan[14] studied the responses of premature infants' parents. They described four tasks that must be accomplished for successful resolution of the crisis of prematurity. These tasks are:

(1)   Anticipatory grief. The mother confronts this task at birth with the possible loss of the baby. The grief response will depend in part on the attachment the mother has established with the baby during pregnancy.

(2)   Facing and acknowledging a feeling of failure for not delivering a normal full-term infant. Substance-abusing mothers may indeed feel a great sense of guilt with a premature birth. This guilt may be expressed as anger and hostility or even withdrawal. The mother struggles with these two tasks until survival of the infant seems secure.

(3)   The resumption of the process of relating to the baby, which previously had been interrupted. The mother has lost the usual opportunity provided by the full-term pregnancy for the development of readiness for the mothering role. Chemically dependent mothers may not develop this readiness despite a full-term pregnancy.

(4)   The challenge of understanding how a premature baby differs from a normal baby in terms of its special needs and growth patterns.

Mothers who do not accomplish these tasks have increased difficulty in achieving healthy outcomes in parenting their children. The nurse's role is particularly important in the last task. Education about the premature infant's behavior and needs is essential. Nurses need to help these parents see **their baby** as a **real** person, and to learn to care for him appropriately.

Several factors make successful parenting difficult for drug-dependent mothers. The first factor that impacts their parenting ability is their own psychosocial difficulties. They themselves may not have had good parenting. They often face social and emotional isolation. Previously established coping mechanisms may prove to be unsuccessful in facing the crisis of premature parenting. Their own dependency needs and low self-esteem make the responsibility of parenting overwhelming.

Attachment to the baby during a long hospitalization in a special care nursery is essential for effective parenting, yet infrequent and unpredicatable visitation patterns may lead to poor mother–infant bonding. When the mothers do visit, they may not be able to relate to the infant as a real person with special needs.

Factors in the premature infant that contribute to poor parenting include the characteristic behavior of these infants. The premature infant's disorganized state, irritability, and poor feeding ability make it difficult for anyone to feel successful at first in parenting these babies. If the infant is going through withdrawal, these problems are intensified. Often, neither the mother nor the infant receive positive reinforcement from the relationship.

Neither is the environment of the special care nursery (SCN) especially conducive to promoting good parenting. The unit is usually bright and noisy, offering little privacy in which to establish relationships.

Nursing Interventions

The first thing the nurse must do is identify and acknowledge his or her own feelings and prejudices concerning chemically dependent mothers. We cannot work as effectively with these mothers and infants if we have hidden negative feelings. A non-judgemental approach in caring for these infants and their families is necessary. If one can view these mothers as having an illness that can be cured, it will go a long way to facilitate effective nursing intervention.

There is an immediate need to promote a sense of trust in the health care provider. This may be more difficult to achieve when the mother is chemically dependent. In order to accomplish this, nurses need to provide consistent care and information to these mothers and provide them with specific guidelines for expected behavior in the SCN. Education about the SCN and the baby's condition should be done upon admission and throughout the hospitalization. This is best accomplished through primary nursing.

Awareness of the mother's perceptions regarding her childbearing experience and her new role is important. The nurse is often the sounding board for these parents. In doing so, we may need to confront these mothers about their behavior and drug use, but we should do so without being moralistic. We need visitation and phone contact from these mothers. Any support person should be encouraged and allowed to visit with the mother. Lastly, these parents need to see that their baby is receiving appropriate professional care.

Promoting attachment to the infant is essential for developing parenting skills. The most important aspect is to personalize and point out the individuality of the infant. Calling the infant by name and describing his behavior is important, so that mothers see their baby as a real person. It is essential that we educate these parents about the behavior of premature infants. Only in this way can they develop realistic expectations about the baby. Time should be spent explaining the SCN, its policies and routines, and in explaining the infant's condition. Again, consistency is key.

Once mother–infant attachment has begun, it can be reinforced by stressing positive parenting skills, emphasizing successful task accomplishments. After assessment of the mother's learning needs, give step-by-step instructions on how to accomplish a specific task and allow adequate time for questions, explanations, and return demonstration. Avoid frustration; intervene before this occurs. Acknowledge that a specific task may be difficult for anyone. Provide positive reinforcement for accomplishing a task, since the baby often can not.

Be patient; repetition of explanations may be necessary. Be **concrete**. When providing printed material or other learning aids, make sure that the material is at a level the mother can understand.

Role modeling of caretaking behavior is especially important for chemically dependent mothers. Since they may be lacking a positive role model in their own mothers, it is even more important that we provide for this. They need to see us talking to the infant, calling him by name, responding appropriately to his cues. By doing so, these mothers will witness appropriate caretaking skills and in doing so be better able to develop positive parenting skills.

Arrange for time for the mothers to give complete care prior to discharge. Rooming-in or other accomodations that allow the mother to care for the infant for twenty-four hours is essential. Only in this way can the mother develop a sense of reality about what caring for her baby means. Plan for discharge well in advance. Appropriate support must be in place prior to discharge. The discharge planner and social worker can help in making the necessary referrals and obtaining the appropriate assistance for these mothers. Specific agencies such as Visiting Nurses Association can become involved in the follow-up plan prior to discharge.

In summary, the goal is to develop positive parenting skills in chemically dependent women. A consistent plan of care needs to be developed and implemented. It is of primary importance to teach these mothers about their babies to develop a sense of attachment. Effective parenting skills take time to develop and can be enhanced by the observation of a positive role model. The role of the nurse is to provide positive, non-judgemental care for these infants and their mothers facilitating a positive outcome.

REFERENCES

1. Cuskey, W.R., PremKeemor, T. and Ligel, L. (1972). Survey of opiate addiction among females in the U.S. between 1950 and 1970. *Publ. Health Rev.*, **1**, 8 – 39
2. Person, P., Retka, R. and Woodward, J. (1977). *A Method for Estimating Heroin Use Prevalence.* (Rockville, MD: National Institute of Drug Abuse)
3. Zelson, C. (1975). Acute management of neonatal addiction, *Addict. Dis.*, **2**, 159 – 68
4. Burt, M. and Glynn, T. (1976). *A Follow-Up Study of Former Clients of New York City's Addiction Services Agency*, Volume II. (Bethesda, Maryland: Burt Associates)
5. Cuskey, W.R., Berger, L.H. and Densen-Berger. (1981). Issues in the treatment of female addiction: a review and critique of the literature. *Women Ment. Health*, **20**, 269 – 95

6. Colten, M. (1977). *A Discipline and Comparative Analyses of Self-Perceptions and Attitudes of Heroin Addicted Women*. (Rockville, MD: National Institute of Drug Abuse)
7. Finnegan, L.P. (ed.) (1978). *Drug Dependence in Pregnancy: Clinical Management of Mother and Child*. (Rockville, MD: National Institute on Drug Abuse)
8. Dyer, E. (1963). Parenthood as a crisis: A restudy. *Marriage Fam. Living*, **25**,(25), 196–206
9. Eintwisle, D. and Doering, S. (1980). *The First Birth*. (Baltimore: John Hopkins University Press)
10. LaRosa, R. and LaRosa, M. (1981). *Transition to Parenthood*. (Beverly Hills:Sage)
11. LeMasters, E. (1957). Parenthood is crisis. *Marriage Fam. Living*, **19**(4), 352–5
12. Russell, C. (1974). Transition to parenthood: problems and gratifications. *J. Marriage Fam.*, **36**(2), 294–301
13. Blackburn, S. and Lowen, L. (1986). Impact of an infant's premature birth on the grandparents and parents. *J. Obstet. Gynecol. Neonat. Nurs.*, **15**(2), 175–8
14. Caplan, G., Mason, E. and Kaplan, D. (1965). Tour studies of the crisis in parents of prematures. *Commun. Ment. Health*, **1**(2), 149–1
15. Jeffcoate, J., Humphrey, E. and Lloyd, J. (1979). Role perception and response to stress in fathers and mothers following preterm delivery. *Soc. Sci. Med.*, **13**, 139–45
16. Tause, M. and Kramer, L. (1983). The effects of premature birth on parents and their relationship. *Devel. Med. Child Neurol.*, **25**, 459–65

4

Drug Addiction and Pregnancy: The Newborn

Loretta P Finnegan

Family Center, a comprehensive outpatient methadone-maintenance treatment program for drug-dependent women in Philadelphia, recognized the special needs and goals of the pregnant addict. The program provides patients and their children with medical, psychiatric and social services as well as a variety of clinical assessments. Comprehensive psychiatric and psychosocial services include evaluation, consultation, referral, crisis intervention, weekly groups, and individual, couple and family counseling. Vocational services, nutritional counseling, and parenting classes are also included in the treatment of the pregnant addict. Treatment plans facilitate the evaluation of pharmacotherapeutic treatment and rehabilitative goals of both the patient and program through the continued process of documenting, monitoring, and critically assessing and revising the pharmacotherapeutic intervention strategies. The program further provides the mother (and the infant) with a continuous, long-acting pure narcotic (methadone) as opposed to the street addict who encounters unpredictable changes in availability and purity of a shorter-acting agent (heroin) which may result in withdrawal or overdose during pregnancy.

As a result of the clinical practices and follow-up research of Family Center over the past seventeen years, a great deal has been learned about the characteristics and needs of drug-dependent women and about the medical and developmental outcome of their children. These findings have been used to improve treatment delivery to pregnant drug-dependent women, to treat most efficaciously the infants undergoing neonatal abstinence, and to make predictive statements regarding the medical and developmental outcome of children born to drug-dependent women. As a result of the clinical and research activities within Family Center as well as the experience of other clinicians involved in the field of perinatal addiction, the following presents the available data on the effects of maternal drug-dependence upon the newborn.

Medical complications and birthweights in infants born to drug-dependent women have been found to be influenced by: (1) the adequacy of prenatal care, (2) the presence of maternal obstetrical or medical complications, and (3) the abuse of multiple drugs by the mother[1]. The problem of infant morbidity becomes particularly apparent when one considers that the majority of drug-dependent women neglect general health care and prenatal care and tend to abuse more than one drug. Medical complications in pregnant drug-dependent women include the following: anemia, hypertension, and infections such as cellulitis, phlebitis, subacute bacterial endocarditis, septicemia, pneumonia (acute and chronic), hepatitis, tetanus, tuberculosis, urinary tract infections and sexually transmitted diseases. Obstetrical complications exaggerate the situation for mother and child and may include: early and late fetal death, infections including amnionitis, chorioamnionitis, septic thrombophlebitis, as well as abruptio placenta, pre-eclampsia, placental insufficiency with intrauterine growth retardation, premature rupture of membranes and postpartum hemorrhage. Women addicted to drugs have a greater chance of having the onset of premature labor.

Drug-addicted women as a group are not homogeneous, and they may present with multiple psychosocial problems. These include: poor self-esteem, periods of serious depression, poverty, legal problems, home-lessness, lack of social supports, loss of children to foster care or to others and ongoing relationships with drug-abusing or alcoholic men who are more often than not physically abusive to them.

A relationship between depression and the placement of children in foster care has been studied. Significantly higher depression scores were present among the drug-abusing women whose children were in foster placement or had been referred to a child welfare agency than women who were raising children. Legal placement of children is a significant factor in depression; however, it is difficult to ascertain whether child placement is an antecedent or consequential variable. Weissman *et al.* also studied depressed but drug-free women and found that, during acute episodes of depression, the women were less involved with their children, had impaired communication, increased friction, lack of affection and greater guilt and resentment[2]. In responding to their children, they were over-protective, irritable, preoccu-pied, withdrawn, emotionally distant and/or rejecting.

In response to the varying symptoms and degree of depression evidenced by Family Center women, the Beck Depression Inventory (BDI) was routinely included as part of the program's intake procedure. Between 1979 and 1984, approximately 250 women were enrolled in Family Center. Of these, a subsample of 149 women completed the BDI. Seventy-five percent of the 149 women reported varying levels of depression, with the following results: 21% had mild depression, 39% were moderately depressed and 15%

were severely depressed. A group of drug-free but pregnant women who also took the Beck Depression Inventory were used as a control population. Comparison between the two groups indicated that far more Family Center women (75%) were suffering from depression than in the control group (50%)[3].

Due to the psychological stresses seen in drug-dependent women, the Profile of Mood States Inventory was administered[4]. This permits women to rate the frequency of various moods they have been experiencing over a period of a week and identifies transient, subjective, affective states. The Profile of Mood States provides a score on six mood factors, as well as a total mood disturbance score. A study was conducted comparing Profile of Mood States scores of a group of pregnant drug-dependent women ($n=25$) versus a group of pregnant, drug-free control women ($n=25$) matched for age and race. The control women were those who attended the regular prenatal clinic. Analysis revealed that the drug-dependent women scored significantly lower than did controls on vigor ($t=2.17$, $p<0.025$) and significantly higher on confusion ($t=2.48$, $p<0.005$) and depression ($t=2.76$, $p<0.005$). There were no differences between drug-dependent and control women in mean fatigue, tension, anger or total scores. The lack of differences on several mood factors implies distinct similarities in the affect of drug-dependent and drug-free pregnant women of lower socioeconomic status. The relatively high levels of confusion and depression among the drug-dependent women may reflect their illicit drug use or may result from their generally chaotic social environment. Such mood states may lead to parental failures evidenced as child neglect or abuse. Prompt social and psychiatric intervention seem warranted as early in the pregnancy as possible[4].

The presence of violence and abuse are pertinent issues in the lives of drug-dependent women. A research study showed that by using an appropriate questionnaire, one could (1) measure episodes and degrees of violence experienced by women, including acts of physical and sexual abuse occurring in childhood or as an adult, and (2) learn if women reporting a history of violence/abuse were more likely to have had children in foster care. Of the 171 women studied, 40% had children in voluntary or involuntary foster placement. Women with a reported history of sexual trauma, particularly if occuring in childhood or repeatedly, were significantly more likely to have children in foster care ($p<0.01$). Women who were physically abused (without sexual trauma) as children and/or adults were less likely to have their children in placement. This study suggests that failure to resolve childhood sexual trauma or coping with the trauma by use of illicit drugs, disrupts the ability of women to parent their own children. Therefore, the effects of violence toward women, particularly when they themselves were children, may have untoward effects upon their own children[5].

INFANT MORBIDITY AND MORTALITY

The majority of medical comlications seen in neonates born to heroin-dependent women result from prematurity. Hypoxia resulting from an unstable intrauterine environment may cause meconium staining and later aspiration pneumonia, which in itself causes a marked morbidity and increased mortality (see Table 4.1).

Table 4.1 Medical complications in infants of drug-dependent women

Asphyxia neonatorum
Respiratory distress syndrome
Pneumonia
Hypoglycemia
Hypocalcemia
Hyperbilirubinemia
Intracranial hemorrhage
Intrauterine growth retardation
Meconium aspiration
Acquired immune deficiency syndrome

An extensive study in Detroit included a review of 830 infants born to opiate-dependent mothers at Hutzel Hospital[6]. In comparison to a control group of 400 infants, infants of the drug-dependent mothers had an increased incidence of low birthweight, small size for gestational age, and low 1- and 5-minute Apgar scores. Significant postnatal problems, excluding neonatal withdrawal, included jaundice, aspiration pneumonia, transient tachypnea, hyaline membrane disease, and congenital malformations. Congenital malformations were as varied in the infants of drug-dependent mothers as they were in control infants. Although the incidence of congenital malformations was greater in the infants of drug-dependent mothers versus the control population studied, the incidence of 2.4% was not greater than that in the general population.

In Philadelphia, we found that morbidity in infants born to drug-dependent women was directly related to the amount of prenatal care as well as to the type of maternal narcotic dependence[7]. Nearly 75% of infants born to 63 heroin addicts who had no prenatal care suffered neonatal morbidity as did 82% of infants born to 78 methadone-dependent women with inadequate care. The incidence of neonatal morbidity was somewhat less, at 69.9% for infants born to methadone-dependent women receiving adequate prenatal care.

Several investigators have noted that infants born to women who use methadone have somewhat higher birthweights than infants born to women using heroin[8-10]. Relating the birthweights of 377 neonates to a history of maternal narcotic usage, analysis by Kandall et al. revealed a highly significant relationship between the first trimester maternal methadone dosage and birthweight[9]. This study showed that methadone may promote fetal growth in a dose-related fashion even after maternal heroin use, whereas heroin itself has been found to cause fetal growth retardation that may persist beyond the period of addiction. In our Philadelphia investigation, concluded in 1977, the infants whose mothers received comprehensive prenatal care had a lower incidence of smaller birthweights, similar in nature to the infants of the control mothers[7]. Of the infants born to the 63 heroin-dependent mothers who received no prenatal care, 47.6% had low birth-weight (under 2500 g). This is in contrast to an 18.8% incidence of low birthweight for the 135 methadone-maintained mothers with good prenatal care.

In a recent study to further investigate the effects of maternal drug use on the development of neonatal complications, infants of drug-dependent women in treatment ($n=61$) and receiving prenatal care were compared to a drug-free comparison group ($n=81$) enrolled in the same prenatal clinic in Philadelphia[11]. Drugs of abuse for the drug-dependent women included both opiates and non-opiates (39%) or non-opiates only (61%). Maternal, intra-partal and neonatal factors were studied. Maternal age and socioeconomic status were studied and were similar in both groups. No differences between groups were found in Apgar scores, maternal gravidity and parity, race and infant sex. Mean birthweight of infants of drug-dependent women was 2959 g and in the comparison group it was 3230 g. Of the 61 infants born to drug-dependent women, 30% required treatment for abstinence. The drug-dependent women had fewer prenatal clinic visits ($p<0.001$) and length of hospital stay for their infants not treated for abstinence was greater ($p<0.001$). No difference was found in the incidence of intrauterine growth retardation between groups. The incidence of apnea, aspiration pneumonia, and hyperbilirubinemia was greater in infants of drug-dependent women; however, the incidence of meconium in amniotic fluid at the time of delivery was similar in both groups. There were four SIDS deaths (7%) in infants born to drug-dependent women. The results of this study suggest that infants born to drug-dependent women in treatment and receiving prenatal care are still at risk for increased morbidity and mortality during the immediate neonatal period and in early infancy. Although 'adequate' in number, prenatal visits did not occur early in pregnancy when complications could have been treated and possibly avoided, but during the third trimester, where the possibilities for prevention and intervention were limited.

Other areas of concern with regard to the infant included the infant's response to the birth process. A study was undertaken to investigate the effects of maternal drug use on neonatal resuscitation. Infants of drug-dependent women ($n = 56$) were compared to a drug-free control group ($n = 63$). Drugs of abuse for the drug-dependent women included opiates and non-opiates (57%) or non-opiates only (43%). Socioeconomic status, gestational age and parity were similar in both groups. A high incidence of low birthweight was seen in the infants born to drug-dependent women; 13 infants versus 7 infants in the control group. Resuscitation was divided into four levels with increasing degrees of complexity: Level I − suction bulb and/or suction catheter only; Level II − oxygen inhalation and/or positive pressure inhalation in addition to suction; Level III − intubation and visualization of the cords in addition to suction and oxygen administration; Level IV − external cardiac massage. Infants born to drug-dependent women had a higher incidence of Level III and Level IV resuscitation. This was found despite the overwhelming number of black infants in the comparison group (black infants are thought to require more intervention, possibly due to lower birthweights and a negative response to perinatal stress). Levels I and II were similarly administered to the two groups of infants. The type of analgesia or anesthesia received by the mothers during the intrapartum course was not related to the level of resuscitation required by the infants. The results of these data suggest that the risk of requiring increased levels of resuscitation at birth is greater for infants born to drug-dependent women. In the application of this data to current practice, medical facilities which provide care for pregnant drug-dependent women should anticipate problems in the delivery room, and establish appropriate emergency procedures in order to provide optimal care for this high-risk population[12].

Infants born to methadone-maintained mothers have been evaluated longtitudinaly with ophthalmological examinations. Forty infants born to drug-dependent mothers were examined shortly before discharge in the newborn nursery and 29 of these infants were examined at 6 months, 12 months and 18 months of age. Seven infants (24%) were diagnosed as having strabismus. Esotropia (convergent deviation) was seen in 3 infants. Mean birthweight for the 7 infants with strabismus was significantly lower than that of the 22 infants without strabismus ($p = 0.05$). The mean methadone dose at the time of delivery for mothers of infants with strabismus was 47 mg/day and for mothers of infants without strabismus it was 39 mg/day. Both groups used other drugs during the pregnancy, including heroin, diazepam, marijuana, amphetamines and nicotine, at least once. The mechanism of this remarkable increased incidence of strabismus (24%) in these infants in comparison to that in the general population (2.8−5.3%) is unknown. However, these data suggest that maternal use of psychoactive agents during pregnancy as well as associated perinatal risk factors may predispose infants to the development of strabismus. These preliminary data should alert clinicians to closely follow all infants prenatally exposed to psychoactive agents with ophthalmological evaluations[13].

Currently, methadone programs are encountering a large number of individuals who are using cocaine as well as opiates. Therefore, the number of infants born to women who abuse cocaine continues to increase. Subjects of a study conducted within our drug treatment program in Philadelphia, included 237 pregnant women: 91 cocaine-using drug-dependent women, 83 non-cocaine using drug-dependent women, and 63 non-drug-dependent women. Both drug-dependent groups were abusing a variety of substances and the majority were on methadone maintenance. The groups were similar for maternal age, socioeconomic status, nicotine use and parity, but different in race. Abruptio placentae occurred in 8% of the cocaine drug-dependent women. Spontaneous abortions, emergency cesarian sections and meconium staining occurred more often in the cocaine drug-dependent women than in either of the other 2 groups. Birthweight and length, head circumference, gestational age, and 1-minute Apgar scores were significantly lower in the infants of cocaine drug-dependent women. No differences existed in the occurrence of congenital anomalies and intracranial hemorrhage. There were more premature deliveries in the cocaine (21%) than in the non-cocaine (11%) and comparison (4%) groups. Mean neonatal abstinence scores, which incorporated 21 physiological and behavioral parameters to quantify symptoms, were lower for the cocaine-exposed infants. Differences were significant with respect to cry, disturbed tremors, increase muscle tone, excoriations, fever, mottling and loose stools. The results of this study suggest that: (1) cocaine in pregnancy adversely effects maternal and fetal outcome, (2) women who use cocaine during pregnancy have a greater incidence of meconium staining, emergency C-section, abruptio placentae, and SGA infants, (3) infants born to women who abuse cocaine have lower birthweight and length, head circumference, gestational age and Apgar scores at 1 and 5 minutes of age, (4) exposure to cocaine *in utero* does not appear to increase the incidence of neonatal abstinence symptomatology[14].

Our most recent evaluation of the perinatal outcome in 196 infants exposed to methadone *in utero* reveals that 12% were premature, there was a 7.7% fetal loss, 8% were term infants with medical complications and 72% were term with no medical complications except neonatal abstinence.

Twenty-five years ago, when medical scientists did not have the techniques to care for high-risk infants, the majority of infants born to opiate-addicted women did not survive. With the advent of new techniques for the care of sick newborns, and specifically for those born prematurely, mortality rates during the past decade have decreased markedly. Incidences in 1973 and 1977 have been reported as 3–4% compared with 94% mortality of untreated infants and 34% of treated infants as reported in 1956[15]. Currently, if we could reduce the use of multiple drugs, especially cocaine, morbidity and mortality could improve even more dramatically.

Moreover, women who are using intravenous drugs must not share needles and should use 'Safe Sex' practices in order to decrease their chances of contracting the human immunodeficiency virus (HIV). Pregnancies should not occur indiscriminantly as before in these women, since many of their infants, if they are HIV positive, will also be at risk for the disease. Moreover, at this time, with no curative measure and no vaccine, mortality in the infants is inevitable.

NEONATAL ABSTINENCE SYNDROME

Onset of withdrawal symptoms in infants exposed to narcotics *in utero* varies from minutes or hours after birth to 2 weeks of age, but the majority of symptoms appear within 72 hours. Many factors influence the onset of abstinence in individual infants, including the type of drugs utilized by the mother, dosage, timing of the dose before delivery, character of labor, type and amount of anesthesia/analgesia given during labor, maturity, nutrition and the presence of intrinsic disease in the infant.

Several types of clinical courses may occur[16]. Withdrawal may be mild and brief, be delayed in onset, have a stepwise increase to severity, be intermittently present, or have a later biphasic course that includes acute withdrawal followed by improvement, with a later onset of subacute withdrawal. More severe withdrawal seems to occur in infants whose mothers have taken large amounts of drugs for a long time. In general, the closer to delivery a mother takes heroin, the greater the delay in onset of withdrawal and the more severe the symptoms in her baby. The maturity of the infant's own metabolic and excretory mechanism plays an important role after delivery. Duration of symptoms can extend from 6 days to 8 weeks, and symptoms of irritability may persist for 3 months or more. During the later period, the infants may have hyperphagia, increased oral drive, sweating, hyperacusis, irregular sleep patterns, loose stools and poor tolerance to holding or to abrupt changes of position and space.

Neonatal abstinence is described by signs and symptoms of central nervous system hyperirritability, gastrointestinal dysfunction, respiratory distress and vague autonomic symptoms that include yawning, sneezing, mottling and fever[1]. Initially, the infants appear only to be restless. Tremors begin when the infants are disturbed, and progress to the point where they occur when the infants are not disturbed. High-pitched cry, increased muscle tone, and further irritability develop. When examined, the infants have increased deep tendon reflexes and an exaggerated Moro reflex. The rooting reflex is increased, and the infants are frequently seen sucking their fists and thumbs. Yet, when feedings are administered, they have extreme difficulty and regurgitate frequently because of uncoordinated and ineffectual sucking and swallowing reflexes. Because of the occurrence of loose stools, decreased intake, and regurgitation, the infants are susceptible to dehydration and electrolyte imbalance.

Excessive nasal secretions with stuffy nose and rapid respirations, sometimes accompanied by retractions, intermittent cyanosis, and irregular respirations, have been seen in the infants undergoing withdrawal[17-19]. If the infant regurgitates, aspirates, and develops pneumonia, severe respiratory embarrassment can often occur. During the first week of life, increased respiratory rates associated with hypocapnia and an increase in blood pH can occur as well. Similar signs and symptoms can also be seen in adults during drug abstinence.

Although the frequency of respiratory distress syndrome increases progressively with decreasing gestational age in premature infants, no respiratory distress syndrome was noted among the 33 premature infants born to heroin-addicted mothers at the Harlem Hospital Center[20]. Newborn infants of opiate-dependent mothers have been found to achieve tissue oxygen unloading comparable to that of a 6-week-old term infant, which suggests that opiates may function as enzyme inducers, which results in increased blood levels of 2,3-disphosphoglycerate and a decrease in oxygen affinity[21].

Sequential pulmonary function studies, performed from birth to 24 hours of age in infants of drug-dependent mothers, show what appears to be a transient decrease in lung compliance and tidal volume when compared with normal, control infants[19]. By 3 days of age, lung compliance and tidal volume returned to normal control levels in spite of persistent tachypnea and abstinence symptomatology.

In order to evaluate brain growth and cerebral ventricular development of infants undergoing abstinence versus those born to a matched group of prenatally drug-free control women, linear array and later, high resolution real-time sector scanning were used[22,23]. Cranial ultrasound examinations were performed during the first 3 days of life and at 1 month in 22 infants with neonatal abstinence syndrome. The results were compared to those obtained in 15 control infants who were not exposed to narcotic drugs *in utero*. Mothers of the drug-exposed infants had been maintained on methadone ($x=41$ mg daily) and many used unknown quantities of heroin, diazepam or amphetamines. The ultrasound images were examined for ventricular configuration, intracranial hemidiameters, area of the thalami, and width of the temporal lobes. At 24 and 72 hours and at 1 month of age, significantly more drug-exposed than control infants had a small lateral (slit-like) ventricular configuration. The intracranial hemidiameter was significantly smaller in the drug-exposed than in the control infants. All cerebral measurements except the right temporal lobe demonstrated significant growth over the first month of life in both groups of infants. In order to further evaluate the effects of psychoactive drugs taken during gestation on the developing nervous system, ultrasound studies of the brain were obtained at 2 and 6 months following birth. The 2- and 6-month images failed to reveal significant differences between drug-exposed and control infants.

Slit-like ventricles may be due to a lack of visualization of fluid space within the ventricles, a diffuse compression of the ventricles bilaterally, or to decreased production or increased reabsorption of cerebrospinal fluid. By means of ancillary examinations (computerized tomography and trans-fontanelle pressure measurements), the pathogenesis of the slit-like ventricles was found to be unrelated to edema or to increased intracranial pressure. Central nervous system irritability seen in neonatal abstinence appears shortly after birth and is frequently manifested for as long as 6 months. The results suggest a relationship between slit-like ventricles and the period of abstinence although the pathogenesis of the abstinence symptomatology was not defined by the ultrasound studies.

In spite of the above objective findings and the potential for concern, differences in ventricular configuration were not reflected in developmental status at 6 months of age. No differences were found in the Bayley Mental Development Index scores between infants with slit-like ventricles and those with normal ventricles ($t = 0.98$, $p > 0.20$). Furthermore, developmental scores for both groups were well within the normal range of development. Slit-like ventricles at birth do not have an adverse effect on development, at least by 6 months of age, even if resumption of normal ventricular configuration has not occurred[24].

Further elicitation of various aspects of neonatal abstinence have been reported previously. The clinical assessment and the treatment aspects will not be delineated here but have been clearly described in 1984 and 1986[25,26].

The majority of infants born to drug-dependent women undergo neonatal abstinence syndrome and often require pharmacotherapy for the treatment of withdrawal symptoms. Phenobarbital, paregoric, and diazepam have been recommended for the treatment of the syndrome. While some investigators have examined the efficacy of these agents in treating neonatal abstinence syndrome, no data regarding the use of specific pharmacologic agents and developmental outcome was available. Therefore, we evaluated 85 infants born to drug-dependent women who were maintained on methadone during pregnancy. Severity of infant withdrawal was assessed with the Neonatal Abstinence Scoring System[25]. Infants who required pharmacotherapy were randomly assigned to one of four treatment regimens: paregoric, phenobarbital (titration), phenobarbital (loading), and diazepam. When treatment was not successful with the assigned agent, one of the other agent(s) was used. At 6 months of age, the developmental status of infants was assessed with the Bayley Scales of Mental Development. Based on NAS treatment, four groups were delineated: (I) paregoric ($n=21$); (II) phenobarbital ($n=17$); (III) more than one agent ($n=31$); and (IV) no treatment ($n=16$). Data for the phenobarbital loading and titration groups were combined since analysis revealed no differences between groups. All infants who initially received diazepam were included in Group III since diazepam as a single agent was not successful. Results of one way analysis of variance revealed no differences in developmental status between groups ($p<0.10, f=0.25$). Scores for all groups were well within the normal range of development. Implications of these findings include: (1) that the severity of withdrawal is not related to developmental outcome when appropriately managed with pharmacotherapy, and (2) that the use of pharmacotherapy does not adversely effect the developmental outcome and may help ameliorate the consequences of neonatal abstinence syndrome[27].

If the physical, psychological and sociological issues of pregnant opiate-dependent women and their children are appropriately addressed, the potential physical and behavioral effects of psychoactive drugs on the mother, her fetus, the newborn and the child may be markedly reduced. The task for clinicians is enormous when contemplating the rehabilitation of such populations, but must be addressed if we are to decrease the inter-generational transmission of the many problems surrounding drug abuse in pregnancy. To ensure a favorable outcome for mother and infant, certain recommendations should be considered if perinatal addiction is evident. These include:

(1) The pregnant woman who abuses drugs must be designated as high risk and warrants specialized care in a perinatal center where she should be provided with comprehensive services including pharmacotherapy for her addiction, when indicated, obstetrical care and psychosocial counseling.

    (a) Pharmacotherapy for the addicted pregnant woman may involve voluntary drug-free therapeutic communities, methadone detoxification (depending on the time in pregnancy when it is requested) or methadone maintenance.

(b)   The pregnant drug-dependent woman should be admitted to a hospital setting where a complete history and physical examination may be accomplished, including laboratory testing to evaluate her overall health status.

(c)   Psychosocial guidance should be provided by experienced counselors who are aware of the medical as well as the social and psychological needs of this population.

(2)   Careful attention must be given to the assessment and managment of the newborn with regard to potential morbidity because of perinatal stresses as well as the onset, progression, and pharmacologic treatment of abstinence.

(a)   Mother/infant attachment should be encouraged prenatally and postpartum. To decrease the possibility of child neglect, special emphasis should be placed on enhancing parenting skills of these women.

(b)   The continued ability of the mother to care for the infant after discharge from the hospital must be assessed by frequent observation in the home and in clinic settings.

(c)   Although the newborn experiencing intrauterine exposure to narcotic agents may appear normal physically, behaviorally and neurologically at the time of birth, one cannot assume that no effect has occurred. The effect of pharmacologic agents may not become apparent until later in development. Therefore, long-term follow-up studies of infants prenatally exposed to pharmacologic agents are extremely important.

REFERENCES

1.   Finnegan, L.P. (ed.) (1978). *Drug Dependence in Pregnancy: Clinical Management of Mother and Child.* A manual for medical professionals and paraprofessionals prepared for the National Institute on Drug Abuse, Service Research Branch, Rockville, Maryland, US Government Printing Office, Washington DC
2.   Weissman, M., Paykel, E. and Klerman, G. (1972). The depressed woman as a mother. *Soc. Psychiatry*, 7, 99-108
3.   Regan, D.O., Rudrauff, M.E. and Finnegan, L.P. (1981). Parenting abilities in drug-dependent women: the negative effect of depression. *Pediatr. Res.*, 15, 90
4.   Regan, D.O., Tunis, S. and Finnegan, L.P. (1983). Psychosocial status of pregnant drug-dependent women: evaluation by the profile of mood states. *Pediatr. Res.*, 17, 93

5. Regan, D.O., Ehrlich, S.M. and Finnegan, L.P. (1985). Sexual violence and placement of children. *Pediatr. Res.*, **19**, 1309
6. Ostrea, E.M. and Chavez, C.J. (1979). Perinatal problems (excluding neonatal withdrawal) in maternal drug addiction: a study of 830 cases. *J. Pediatr.*, **94**, 292–5
7. Connaughton, J.F., Reeser, D., Schut, J. and Finnegan, L.P. (1977). Perinatal addiction: outcome and management. *Am. J. Obstet. Gynecol.*, **129**, 679–86
8. Connaughton, J.F., Finnegan, L.P., Schut, J. and Emich. J.P. (1975). Current concepts in the management of the pregnant opiate addict. *Addict. Dis.*, **2**, 21–35
9. Kandall, S.R., Albin, S., Lowinson, J., Berle, B., Eidelman, A.I. and Gartner, L.M. (1976). Differential effects of maternal heroin and methadone use on birthweight. *Pediatrics*, **58**, 681–5
10. Zelson, C. (1973). Infant of the addicted mother. *N. Engl. J. Med.*, **288**, 1393–5
11. Berger, B., Ehrlich, S.M. and Finnegan, L.P. (1986). Morbidity and mortality of infants born to drug-dependent women. *Pediatr. Res.*, **20**, 1286
12. Berger, B., Ehrlich, S.M., Matteucci, T. and Finnegan, L.P. (1986). Intrapartum resuscitation of infants born to drug-dependent women. In: Harris, L.S. (ed.) *Problems of Drug Dependence*, National Institute on Drug Abuse Monograph Series 67. U.S. Government Printing Office
13. Nelson, L.B., Ehrlich, S.M., Calhoun, J.H., Matteucci, T. and Finnegan, L.P. (1987). The occurrence of strabismus in infants prenatally exposed to psychoactive drugs. *Am. J. Dis. Child.*, **141**, 175–8
14. Livesay, S., Ehrlich, S.M. and Finnegan, L.P. (1987). Cocaine and pregnancy: Maternal and infant outcome. *Pediatr. Res.*, **21**, 387
15. Goodfriend, M.J., Shey, I.A. and Klein, M.D. (1956). The effects of maternal narcotic addiction on the newborn. *Am. J. Obstet. Gynecol.*, **71**, 29–36
16. Desmond, M.M. and Wilson, G.S. (1975). Neonatal abstinence syndrome, recognition and diagnosis. *Addict. Dis.*, **2**, 113–21
17. Glass, L., Rajegowda, B.K. and Kahn, E.J. (1972). Effect of heroin withdrawal on respiratory rate and acid–base status in the newborn. *N. Engl. J. Med.*, **286**, 746–8
18. Klain, D.B., Krauss, A.N. and Auld, P.A.M. (1972). Tachypnea and alkalosis in infants of narcotic addicted mothers. *NY State J. Med.*, **72**, 367–8
19. Lin, T.H., Finnegan, L.P., Reeser, D.S., Shaffer, T.H. and Delivoria-Papadopoulus, M. (1979). Sequential pulmonary function studies of drug-dependent infants since birth. *Acta Paediatr. Sin.*, **20**, 73–9
20. Glass, L., Ragegowda, B.K. and Evans, H.E. (1971). Absence of respiratory distress syndrome in premature infants of heroin-addicted mothers. *Lancet*, **2**, 265
21. Finnegan, L.P., Schouraie, Z., Emich, J.P., Connaughton, J.R., Schut, J. and Delivoria-Papadopoulous, M. (1974). Alterations of the oxygen hemoglobin equilibrium curve and red cell, 2,3-disphosphoglycerate in cord blood of infants born to narcotic addicted mothers. *Pediatr. Res.*, **8**, 344
22. Pasto, M.E., Graziani, L.J., Tunis, S.L., Dealing, J.M., Kurtz, A.B. and Finnegan, L.P. (1985). Ventricular configuration and cerebral growth in infants born to drug-dependent mothers. *Pediatr. Radiol.*, **15**, 77–81
23. Pasto, M.E., Ehrlich, S.M., Deiling, J. and Finnegan, L.P. (1986). The effect of narcotics in-utero on infant brain growth. A cross-secional study. *Pediatr. Res.*, **20**, 1075
24. Kaltenbach, K., Pasto, M., Graziani, L. and Finnegan, L.P. (1985). Early neurodevelopment in infants with slit-like ventricles. *Pediatr. Res.*, **19**, 1297
25. Finnegan, L.P. (1984). Neonatal abstinence. In Nelson, N. (ed.) *Current Therapy in Neonatal–Perinatal Medicine*, pp. 262–270. (Ontario, Canada: BC Decker, Inc.)
26. Finnegan, L.P. (1986). Neonatal abstinence syndrome: assessment and pharmacotherapy. In Rubaltelli, F.F. and Granati, B. (eds.) *Neonatal Therapy: An Update*, pp. 122–146. (Amsterdam–New York–Oxford: Excerpta Medica)
27. Kaltenbach, K. and Finnegan, L.P. (1986). Neonatal abstinence, pharmacotherapy, and the developmental outcome. *Neurobehav. Toxicol. Teratol.*, **8**, 353–5

5

Marijuana and Cigarette Smoking during Pregnancy: Neonatal Effects

Barry Zuckerman

INTRODUCTION

Tobacco and marijuana are commonly inhaled substances which when consumed during pregnancy raise questions and concerns regarding their impact on fetal growth and development. While the information regarding the impact of cigarette smoking on the newborn has been well studied for over twenty years and has consistently been associated with 150 to 250 g decrease in average birthweight and other neonatal effects, the evidence regarding marijuana use and birthweight is limited and inconsistent. This chapter presents what is known about teratogenicity of cigarette and marijuana smoking. Teratogenicity refers to the ability of a drug consumed in pregnancy to cause a birth defect or other adverse fetal outcome. While teratogenetic effects have traditionally been associated with major structural defects, such as those seen with thalidomide, intrauterine growth retardation (IUGR) and neurobehavioral dysfunction may be more common and sensitive effects of drugs consumed during pregnancy. This is clearly the case with cigarette smoking and marijuana where structural defects have not been documented. This review will also attempt to explain the inconsistencies in findings associated with the teratogenicity of marijuana use.

MARIJUANA

Marijuana use is most common among individuals in their late teens and early twenties. The range of women reported to use marijuana during pregnancy varies from 5% to 34%[1-8]. Variability of reported use among studies may be due to different populations being studied, different assessment protocols, secular changes in use or reporting bias. Since many fetuses appear to be exposed to marijuana *in utero*, it is important to ascertain whether they will experience any adverse effects from this exposure.

Pharmacology

Marijuana is the name given to flowering tops from the plant *Cannabis sativa*. More than 400 chemicals have been identified in the cannabis plant[9]. The principal psychoactive ingredient in marijuana is 1,9-tetrahydro-cannabinol (9-THC). The main route of administration of marijuana in humans is by inhalation. More than one-half the 9-THC present in a marijuana cigarette is absorbed[10]. 9-THC has a high affinity for lipids and therefore accumulates in fatty tissues throughout the body[11]. A single dose of cannabis in humans takes as much as 30 days to be excreted with a half-life in tissues of about 7 days[12]. Most of the 9-THC is metabolized in the liver and eliminated in the feces. Studies with laboratory animals demonstrate that marijuana inhibits the secretion of reproductive hormones (luteinizing hormone, follicle-stimulating hormone and prolactin). However, with chronic drug exposure, tolerance develops to many of these inhibiting effects, probably reflecting adaptation of neural mechanisms in the hypothalamus[13]. Studies in humans confirm the development of tolerance with a return to normal hormone concentration in young women who regularly use marijuana[14]. The development of tolerance may be a factor in explaining some of the conflicting data in human and animal studies.

In addition, similar to cigarettes, marijuana produces increased carbon monoxide levels in the blood resulting in hypoxia[15]. In addition to these indirect effects, marijuana may have a direct effect on the fetus since it crosses the placenta. Placental transfer is higher in early pregnancy than in late pregnancy[16].

Studies in Animals

The animal literature on the effects of maternal marijuana exposure during pregnancy has recently been summarized by Abel[17]. Malformations are not consistently observed and usually occur only at high marijuana levels obtained by intraperitoneal administration. An appropriate inhalation model has not yet been developed. Intrauterine growth retardation is observed in many animal studies. However, this may be explained by a decrease in food and water consumption associated with marijuana use[18]. In a study comparing offspring of pregnant rats orally administered 9-THC with pair-fed and watered controls, the marijuana-treated rats exhibited a significant dose-related decrease in pregnancies carried to term, a decrease in weight gain during pregnancy, and lower birthweight[19]. However, in one study, an enriched protein diet prevented marijuana-induced developmental problems, such as delayed onset of the righting reflex, eye opening, and visual placing[20]. Thus, good nutrition may protect against adverse effects of marijuana exposure during pregnancy.

A possible synergistic effect of marijuana and alcohol has recently been demonstrated[21]. In two different species, marijuana plus alcohol caused a significant increase in fetal mortality, whereas the fetal mortality for either drug alone did not differ from pair-fed controls. Thus, the combination of two commonly used drugs has a greater negative impact than that associated with either drug alone.

In studies assessing chromosome damage in cells of animals, no effects are demonstrated when cells are incubated with 9-THC[22]. This finding is consistent with studies in human subjects[23].

Studies in Humans

Growth and Physical Development

Epidemiologic data concerning the effects on fetal development of marijuana use during pregnancy among humans are limited and inconsistent. Greenland et al.[24] compared 35 regular marijuana users with 35 non-users matched by age, ethnicity, parity, and center of care. Each subject's drug use history was supplemented by laboratory determinations of urine canabinoids. Significantly, more marijuana users exhibited precipitous labor and their infants were significantly more likely to exhibit meconium staining (25% vs. 5%). Statistical adjustment for other risk factors, e.g. income, smoking, alcohol use, and time of first prenatal visit, did not alter results. The percentage of subjects with precipitous labor and meconium staining increased proportionally to the reported frequency of marijuana use. Although not significant, marijuana users exhibited higher levels of anemia, poor weight gain, suspected IUGR, and prolonged or arrested labor.

Tennes and Blackard[25] examined 278 offspring of mothers interviewed before and after delivery at two public hospital outpatient obstetric clinics. Infant outcomes were obtained from the infants' medical records. When confounding variables were controlled statistically, marijuana use was not associated with shorter duration of gestation, low infant birthweight, decreased length or congenital anomalies. It is possible that clinically meaningful relationships did not produce statistical significance in this and the previous study because of the small sample size.

Only six studies of humans have examined samples of sufficient size to adequately control for potential confounding effects of other maternal habits, such as smoking, drinking, or other illicit drug use. In a subsequent study with a larger sample size, Tennes et al. investigated 756 mother–infant pairs of

75

whom 34% used marijuana during pregnancy[5]. Infant birth length was the only measure influenced by marijuana when confounding variables were taken into account. Smoking three joints per day was associated with a reduction of 0.55 centimeters in length. This reduction in length was approximately comparable to that attributable to smoking one and half packs per day of cigarettes. Finally, marijuana use during pregnancy was independently associated with a prolongation of gestation. No association between marijuana use and Apgar scores, neonatal medical complications or congenital anomalies were seen.

In a study of 583 women who were interviewed during the prenatal period and after delivery, Fried et al.[2] observed a statistically significant reduction of 0.8 weeks gestation among offspring of mothers who smoked six or more marijuana joints per week during pregnancy even when effects of cigarette smoking, alcohol use, parity, mother's prepregnancy weight, and sex of the infant were controlled analytically. When these confounding variables were controlled, infants of these heavy marijuana users were 78 g lighter than the infants of non-users. This difference was not statistically significant. In the subsample of subjects from this study, Fried compared the infants of 25 marijuana-using women to the infants of 25 matched controls for the presence of minor physical anomalies. The results of this investigation did not show any association between anomalies and marijuana use during pregnancy[26].

Linn et al.[3], at the Boston Hospital for Women, interviewed the largest number of women to date. Of 17,136 women who delivered at the hospital between August 1977 and March 1980, 12,718 women were interviewed shortly after delivery. Infant outcomes were obtained from the infant records. Women were asked whether they used marijuana during pregnancy and, if so, whether they used it on an occasional, weekly, or daily basis. When confounding variables were controlled, no independent association was observed between marijuana use and gestation of less than 37 weeks or birth weight below 2500 g. An odds ratio of 1.36 was observed between the use of marijuana and infants having major malformations. This relationship was suggestive but did not reach statistical significance at $p < 0.05$.

A study of 1690 mother–child pairs at Boston City Hospital by Hingson et al.[1] compared infants of 234 mothers who reported marijuana use during pregnancy to the infants of non-users. Other maternal characteristics that might influence fetal growth and development, such as cigarette smoking, maternal drinking, weight gain during pregnancy, maternal height, pre-pregnancy weight, and medical history, were controlled analytically. Marijuana use was found to be independently associated with lower infant birthweight and decreased length. Women who used marijuana less than three times per week during pregnancy delivered infants 95 g smaller than infants of non-users, and women who used marijuana three or more times per week delivered babies 139 g smaller than infants of non-users. In comparison, women who smoked one pack or more of cigarettes daily delivered infants 83 g smaller than did non-users.

The same study did not identify significant independent associations between maternal marijuana use and shorter duration of gestation, presence of congenital malformation, or lower one or five minute Apgar scores. The study found, however, that among a variety of maternal habits and characteristics, maternal marijuana use was the strongest independent predictor of whether a mother delivered an infant with a combination of anomalies considered compatible with fetal alcohol syndrome. This finding underlines the possibility that marijuana use may contribute independently to the development of abnormalities heretofore thought to be exclusively caused by excessive alcohol use during pregnancy. It is also possible that interactions among substances may occur that are detrimental to fetal growth similar to the synergistic effect of alcohol and marijuana for animals reported by Abel[21].

Another large sample of 7310 births was studied by Gibson et al.[4]. Mothers of the infants were interviewed extensively during both the prenatal and postnatal periods about their health and health habits. Marijuana use was classified as non-user, up to once a week, and more than once a week. Five percent of women smoked marijuana during pregnancy; of these only 5% used it habitually. Marijuana users were significantly more likely to deliver premature infants even when parity, maternal age, alcohol and tobacco use were controlled analytically. Among women who used marijuana once a week, 25% reported low birthweight ($p < 0.05$) but this relationship was not found when only full-term infants were examined. No significant independent relationship were observed between marijuana use and low Apgar scores, congenital malformations, or perinatal death.

Finally, a recent study[8] of 3,857 pregnancies in New Haven, Connecticut, demonstrated that regular use of marijuana (at least 2-3 times monthly) among whites was associated with an odds ratio of 2.6 for delivering a low birthweight infant, 1.9 for a premature infant, and 2.3 for a small for gestational age infant after adjustment for other factors. These odds ratios represent statistically significant elevations except for the increase in prematurity which is of borderline significance. Non-white marijuana users were not at further increased risk for delivering a low birthweight or small for gestational age infant beyond the elevated rates of these conditions already experienced by non-whites in general. An interaction between ethnicity and marijuana use to infant birthweight has also been described in a subsequent analysis of the sample studied by Hingson et al.[1]. Amaro et al.[27] demonstrated that after controlling for other confounding variables, the mean birthweight for infants of mothers who used marijuana prior to and during pregnancy compared to mothers of infants who had never smoked marijuana was 350 g lower for Hispanics, 255 g lower for other blacks, 60 g lower for American blacks and 40 g lower for whites. While these two studies show an interaction between the association between marijuana use and ethnicity in contributing to birthweight, the direction of the relationship is different for whites and non-whites in the two studies. While the studies defined ethnic groups differently, there is a common pattern in both studies that helps explain the findings. The effect of marijuana use on lowering birthweight was found only in the groups in each sample with a low incidence of marijuana use. In Amaro's study[27], marijuana use among Hispanics and other blacks was rare, while in the Hatch and Bracken (1986) study[8], marijuana use was rare among whites. It is possible that the social acceptability associated with marijuana use is different among ethnic groups in different geographic areas or study populations. When it occurs frequently it may be acceptable behavior, while in other groups who use it less frequently, it is a deviant behavior. It is possible that in Amaro's study the Hispanic and other black women and in the Hatch and Bracken study the white women who use marijuana during pregnancy represent a very different and perhaps a more at-risk subset within the study population than the other women who smoke marijuana during pregnancy. A pattern of greater deviancy among Hispanic women who use other psychoactive drugs (e.g. narcotics) has been reported[28]. Therefore, marijuana use among subpopulations who are less likely to use the drug may represent a marker for other risk factors associated with low birthweight. In each case the effect being attributed to marijuana may actually be due to a more complex set of factors which are not accounted for in the analysis. Therefore, it may not be marijuana use *per se* that is associated with birthweight, but rather that when marijuana use is a socially aberrant behavior, it may be associated with other at risk behaviors not measured in either study. This suggests that it is important to understand the social context of marijuana use since in some groups use may be associated with other risk factors related to low birthweight, while in other groups it may not have the same associations.

The inconsistent results of studies investigating the relationship between marijuana use during pregnancy and birthweight are highlighted in a recent paper investigating two prospectively studied groups of approximately 1400 pregnant women per group[7]. The subjects were obtained from three New York city hospitals. The first group consisted of women interviewed between June 1975 and March 1981. The second group was interviewed with a slightly different questionnaire between August 1979 and October 1983. The women in each group are considered as independent samples because of the use of different questionnaires. The association of marijuana use with birthweight was not consistent between the two groups reported in this study. For women in Group 1, marijuana use two to four times per month was associated with a significant increase in average birthweight while both more and less frequent use did not demonstrate any trend or significant effects. In contrast, for women in Group 2, marijuana use greater than two times per week demonstrated a decrease in birthweight with increase in frequency of marijuana use when confounding variables were controlled. A similar type of analysis was conducted for alcohol use and cigarette smoking during pregnancy. The impact of cigarette smoking on birthweight was consistent in both phases of the study while the impact of alcohol on birthweight was inconsistent between Group 1 and Group 2 of the study similar to marijuana. The results of this study representing two cohorts reflects the findings in the literature; the relationship between marijuana use during pregnancy and birthweight is inconsistent while the relationship between cigarette smoking and birthweight is consistent.

The inconsistent results in research regarding the association between marijuana use and birthweight may be explained by a number of factors. It is possible that the composition of marijuana varies over time and geographic areas or that the content of the marijuana varies due to the presence or absence of contaminants or herbicides. Difference in the effects of marijuana use might also be due to changes over time or in different geographic areas in the use of other interrelated drugs. Methodologic differences such as prospective or retrospective ascertainment of drug use, small and varying percentage of heavy users and incomplete control of confounding variables among studies may also account for differences in the results of studies.

Another possible methodologic reason for the inconsistency in results is a reliance by these studies on maternal self-report of marijuana use, cigarette smoking and drinking with disproportionate underreporting by different study populations. This is especially important when the independent variables such as marijuana, alcohol or cigarette use are highly interrelated. Maternal marijuana use during pregnancy in particular may be under-reported relative to cigarette and alcohol use because marijuana is illegal. In order to assess the validity of self-reported marijuana use during pregnancy, Hingson and colleagues randomly allocated pregnant women into a group who were told their urine would be tested for marijuana, alcohol and other drugs and another group not so tested[29]. The women told that they would be tested reported more marijuana use during pregnancy than did untested women. Moreover, urine assays identified more women who used marijuana during pregnancy than were willing to admit it in the interview even after being told their urine would be tested. No differences in reported drinking or cigarette smoking during pregnancy were found between urine tested and untested women. This finding of underreporting was further supported by the same research group in a larger study[6]. In this study, 15% of the total number of marijuana users during pregnancy denied use but had a positive urine assay for marijuana metabolites during pregnancy. Urines were analyzed twice during pregnancy. It is however possible that some individuals with positive urines who denied use were passively exposed to marijuana. A recent study demonstrates that with sufficient time of high marijuana exposure urinary metabolites of marijuana can be detected, as well as subjects experiencing subjective effects[30]. If marijuana has a negative effect on birthweight, it is unlikely that passive exposure is any less detrimental than active exposure at similar blood levels.

Cocaine is not absorbed by passive exposure and the numbers of women who underreported cocaine in this study[6] was even higher. Of all cocaine users in the same study sample, 26% had positive urines for cocaine metabolites and had previously denied use during the questionnaire. These findings raise concerns about conclusions that may have been reached on studies on fetal outcome that rely entirely on maternal self-report on marijuana, alcohol and cigarette use in pregnancy. If marijuana use is underreported relative to alcohol and cigarettes as this study suggests, it is possible that potentially adverse effects of marijuana may be inadvertently misattributed to alcohol or nicotine. It is also possible that potentially interactive effects of marijuana with alcohol, tobacco or other drugs have not been adequately examined.

On balance, the literature based on human studies of the possible effects of marijuana and fetal development is limited and inconsistent. Only five studies have reported the possible independent relationship between marijuana use and adverse fetal outcome in samples of more than 1,000 mother–child pairs[1,3,4,7,8]. Since the fetal outcome affected by marijuana use varied among studies, no firm conclusions can be drawn. Finally, of these five studies, none used a biologic marker to confirm the validity of self-report on marijuana.

Neurobehavioral Functioning

Limited information is available regarding the impact of marijuana use during pregnancy on the neurobehavioral functioning of newborns. In the study by Tennes et al.[5], marijuana was not associated with any of the individual items on the Brazelton Neonatal Behavioral Assessment Scale nor to scores on clusters of the Brazelton items when confounding variables were controlled. Contrary to this finding using the same assessment (Brazelton Neonatal Behavioral Assessment Scale) Fried demonstrated that more newborns of heavy marijuana smokers either did not respond to a light stimulus or did not habituate to it. In addition, the newborns of the marijuana smokers demonstrated more tremors and startles in addition to being less successful at self-quieting. By thirty days post-delivery there did not appear to be any differences between the infants of marijuana users and those of non-users[31].

In a follow-up report by the same author using a larger sample size, regular marijuana use during pregnancy (one or more joints per week) among 24 women (9.6% of the study population) was associated with increased startles, increased tremors and decreased ability to habituate to a light stimulus among their infants on approximately day 3 of life compared to infants whose mothers did not use marijuana or who were light users (less than one joint per week). Confounding variables such as gestational age, age at testing, family income, maternal age, caffeine, other drug use (alcohol and cigarettes) and obstetric medications were controlled statistically.

As part of the same study population, Fried examined the neurologic status of 9- and 30-day-old infants by using the Prechtl Neurological Examination[33]. This examination consists of two general components: (1) observation of the infant's state, resting posture and movements, and (2) elicited reflexes and responses. Compared to the infrequent or non-users of marijuana, infants of marijuana users demonstrated increased startles and tremors (associated with the Moro reflex) at both 9 and 30 days. In addition, infants of marijuana users had poor hand to mouth activity at 9 days, increased elbow resistance and forearm recoil and Babinski reflex at 30 days. The increased tremors and startles at 9 and 30 days are consistent with results of the Brazelton Assessment among the 3-day-old newborns.

While the magnitude of marijuana effects is small, the findings raise concern that marijuana use during pregnancy may affect newborn neurobehavioral functioning. It is important to recognize that the low-risk population under study enhanced the likelihood of detecting subtle effects of drugs. Regardless, this effect may have future implications for later functioning by indicating a small but fixed neurological dysfunction and/or have a negative impact on mother–infant interaction.

Summary

Most of the available information demonstrates an association between marijuana use and some adverse neonatal outcome. However, the lack of consistency in specific effects suggests considerable caution before ascribing pregnancy risk to maternal marijuana use. Clearly, more research must be conducted before any firm conclusions can be reached. Since underreporting of marijuana use during pregnancy has been reported, laboratory verification of self-report should be part of the research design.

CIGARETTE SMOKING

In 1957, Simpson[34] demonstrated that cigarette smoking during pregnancy was associated with lower birthweight and that the more cigarettes smoked, the greater the decrease in birthweight. Subsequent studies have confirmed this relationship and have linked cigarette smoking during pregnancy with other adverse fetal and neonatal outcomes. In spite of this information, smoking during pregnancy continues. A survey conducted in 1977 demonstrates that only 35% of women smokers stopped smoking during pregnancy, while another 32% decreased their amount of smoking[35].

Pharmacology

Cigarette smoke contains more than 2000 pharmacologically active substances[36]. Most of these chemical agents are in the gas phase of cigarette smoke and include carbon monoxide, nitrous oxide, cyanide, and other compounds. Only a small number of these compounds, such as nicotine and hydrocarbon products, are found in the particulate phase of cigarette smoke.

Nicotine is the most studied substance and is considered the compound primarily responsible for the pharmacologic effects of smoking. Nicotine is readily absorbed by the lungs. Blood nicotine levels vary according to the duration and intensity of inhalation, number of inhalations per cigarette, brand of cigarette, and the presence or absence of filters. Nicotine is water and lipid soluble and is rapidly distributed throughout the body. It is metabolized by the liver, kidneys, and lungs, into two main metabolites: cotinine and nicotine-1-N-oxide and is primarily eliminated by the kidneys. Fifty percent is eliminated during the first 2 h after smoking a cigarette, and 25% more of the drug is eliminated over the subsequent 22 h.

While nicotine is known to cross the placenta[17], the effects of nicotine on the fetus are primarily indirect through maternal vasoconstriction and reduced oxygen availability. For example, nicotine stimulates the release of catecholamines from peripheral nerve cells and adrenal glands. In a study of eight chronic smokers at 34 weeks gestation, Quigley et al.[37] demonstrated increased levels of norepinephrine and epinephrine within 2.5 min of smoking a cigarette resulting in an increase in maternal pulse and blood pressure followed by an increase in fetal heart rate.

Cigarette smoke also contains carbon monoxide which combines with hemoglobin to form carboxyhemoglobin in a smoking mother and her fetus. The levels of carboxyhemoglobin may be 3–8 times higher than normal thus impairing oxygenation[38]. Both of these mechanisms cause fetal hypoxia and are probably additive in their contribution to decreasing the birthweight of the fetus. These and other mechanisms[38] may be responsible for adverse fetal effects attributed to cigarette smoking.

Studies in Animals

Animal studies generally agree with the human epidemiologic findings associating cigarette smoking with low birthweight, spontaneous abortion, and behavioral dysfunction[17]. Malformations are seldom seen except at high doses of nicotine, which are usually injected intraperitoneally or subcutaneously. Inhalation models for animals have not been well developed at this time.

Studies in Humans

Spontaneous Abortion

The relationship between cigarette smoking and spontaneous abortion has been documented in numerous studies. When other risk factors are controlled, women who smoke cigarettes during pregnancy are 1.2 – 1.8 times more likely to have a spontaneous abortion as those who do not smoke[39,40]. The mechanism for this epidemiologic association has not been identified but might include abnormalities in placental development or dysfunction in hormones that sustain pregnancy, such as progesterone or prolactin.

Sudden Infant Death Syndrome

A case – control study demonstrated that mothers of victims of sudden infant death syndrome (SIDS) were more likely to smoke cigarettes either during pregnancy or after their baby was born[41]. Two studies in which data were prospectively collected also demonstrate that maternal cigarette smoking significantly increases the likelihood of SIDS[42,43].

Apgar Scores

Three studies have indicated that maternal cigarette smoking during pregnancy is associated with low Apgar scores[45,46]. These studies do not assess whether cigarette smoking or other factors during pregnancy contribute to lower Apgar scores when obstetric, labor, and delivery risks are controlled analytically. When these potentially confounding factors were controlled in a study of 1709 mother – child pairs at Boston City Hospital, no significant independent association was demonstrated between cigarette smoking and Apgar scores[47].

Fetal Growth and Physical Development

Studies assessing the association between cigarette smoking during pregnancy and birthweight consistently demonstrate a decrease in birthweight as well as an increased percentage of low-birthweight infants (2500 g or less). In addition, a dose-related response between the number of cigarettes smoked and decrease in birthweight as well as the percentage of low-birthweight infants is demonstrated. Abel[17] summarizes the effect of cigarette smoking on birthweight. The babies of smokers have reductions in birthweight from 40 to 430 g, with an average weight reduction of about 200 g as compared with the birthweights of non-smokers. These findings remain consistent when numerous variables are controlled. For white mothers, the incidence of low-birthweight babies ranges from 4.8% for women who do not smoke, to 8% for women who smoke 1 – 10 cigarettes per day, to 13.4% for women who smoke more than 20 cigarettes per day. For black women, the incidence of low-birthweight babies ranges from 8.3% for women who do not smoke, to 13.6% for women who smoke 1 – 10 cigarettes per day, to 22.7% for women who smoke more than 20 cigarettes per day. A recent study demonstrated serum cotinine (the major metabolite of nicotine) levels were more strongly correlated with reduced birthweight than with smoking history. Smokers of more than 25 cigarettes per day (2.7% of sample) had infants 289 g lighter than non-smokers, while women with cotinine levels of greater than 28 ng/ml (also 2.7% of sample) had infants that were 441 g lighter[48]. This study supports the importance of using biochemical markers of cigarette smoking and other substances in studies of pregnancy outcome. Studies comparing infant birthweights show that mothers who quit smoking during pregnancy have babies with higher birthweights than do mothers who continue to smoke during pregnancy[22]. A randomized clinical trial of counseling intervention demonstrated its effectiveness in reducing smoking during pregnancy[22]. Another randomized clinical trial of counseling intervention also demonstrated its effectiveness in reducing smoking and increasing birthweight and length[49].

While smoking during pregnancy decreases growth, the nature of the growth deficit in terms of newborn body composition has only been recently assessed[50]. Anthropometric indices of subcutaneous fat deposition and lean body mass were assessed in infants of 109 smokers and 176 non-smokers.

Whereas birthweight, length and head circumference were smaller for infants of smoking mothers, there was no difference between the two groups of infants in any of the skinfold measurements or in the calculated cross-sectional fat area of the upper arm. These new data suggest that the reduction in birthweight of infants whose mothers smoke is due primarily to a decrease in the lean body mass of the newborn, while deposition of subcutaneous fat is relatively unaffected. In addition to decreased birthweight, babies of mothers who smoke have been shown in some studies to have decreased birth length[51] and decreased head circumference[52].

The results of studies assessing the association between cigarette smoking during pregnancy and congenital malformations are conflicting. The British Perinatal Mortality Survey ($n = 17,418$) demonstrated that maternal smoking was associated with congenital heart defects, even when age, parity, and social class were controlled[53]. The United States Collaborative Perinatal Project ($n = 50,282$) did not demonstrate this association[54]. In the US study, the total number of malformed babies was unrelated to maternal smoking. However, several categories of malformations did demonstrate a somewhat increased relative risk for children of women who smoke during pregnancy, including malformations of the CNS, hypospadias, inguinal hernia, and eye and ear malformations. A third study ($n = 18,631$) demonstrated increased risk of cleft palate and/or cleft lip in infants of mothers who smoked during pregnancy[55]. Other studies report no association between congenital malformations and maternal smoking[56-58]. These studies have smaller sample sizes than the previous studies, which could account for the lack of a positive relationship. However, the lack of reported consistent malformations or pattern of malformations suggests that cigarette smoking may not by itself cause malformations.

Neurobehavioral Effects

The impact of cigarette smoking during pregnancy on newborn behavior and on later child development has been assessed. On the Brazelton Neonatal Behavioral Assessment Scale (BNBAS) newborns of mothers who smoked during pregnancy performed less well on items such as habituating to sound or orienting to a voice as compared with newborns whose mothers did not smoke[59]. This study did not control for other drugs, such as alcohol or marijuana.

Another study found that newborns exposed *in utero* to greater amounts of alcohol and nicotine performed less well on two operant conditioning tasks: head turning and sucking[60]. Landesman-Dwyer *et al.*[61] observed that newborns of heavier smoking and drinking women coughed and sneezed more and were less visually alert. Other studies have demonstrated more crying[62] and poorer autonomic regulations as demonstrated by more tremors and startles and increased lability of skin color[63].

These studies do not demonstrate a clinically significant impact on neonatal behavior that can be independently attributed to cigarette smoking. Because of the difficulty in identifying newborns who are only exposed to cigarette smoking and not to other factors that would affect their behavior, it is unlikely that clinically important differences will be demonstrated. If there are differences, however, current research indicates that they will be small.

Long-term follow-up evaluation of children's cognitive and developmental functioning seems to indicate that, when sociodemographic factors are controlled, children exposed to cigarette smoking *in utero* do less well on tests of cognitive, psychomotor, language, and general academic achievement, including reading and mathematics. Whereas differences are statistically significant between children exposed to cigarette smoking *in utero* versus children who are not, differences are small compared with other factors that affect children's performance[64,65].

Summary

Cigarette smoking during pregnancy is associated with lower birthweights presumably due to fetal hypoxia. A higher incidence of spontaneous abortions and SIDS is also documented. While cigarette smoking appears to have a small effect on neurobehavioral functioning, its effect on later development raises important questions about the effect seen in the newborn period. Does the neonatal neurobehavioral dysfunction have a negative impact on mother–infant interaction and/or represent a small but fixed neurological dysfunction? There is no stong evidence linking cigarettes with congenital malformations or lower Apgar scores.

ACKNOWLEDGEMENTS

This work was supported by a grant from the National Institute of Drug Abuse (R01DA03508). I thank Howard Bauchner, MD, for his helpful comments and Ms Jeanne McCarthy for her help in preparing the manuscript.

REFERENCES

1. Hingson, R., Alpert, J., Day, N., Dooling, E., Kayne, H., Morelock, S., Oppenheimer, E., Rosett, H., Weiner, L. and Zuckerman, B.S. (1982). Effects of maternal drinking and marijuana use on fetal growth and development. *Pediatrics*, **70**, 539

2. Fried, P.A., Watkinson, B. and Willan, A. (1984). Marijuana use during pregnancy and decreased length of gestation. *Am. J. Obstet. Gynecol.*, **150**, 23

3. Linn, S., Schienbaum, S., Monson, R., Rosner, R., Stubblefield, P.C. and Ryan, K.J. (1984). The association of marijuana use with outcome of pregnancy. *Am. J. Public Health*, **73**, 1161

4. Gibson, G.T., Bayhurst, P.A. and Colley, D.P. (1983). Maternal alcohol, tobacco and cannabis consumption and the outcome of pregnancy. *Aust. N.Z. Obstet. Gynecol.*, **23**, 16

5. Tennes, K., Avitable, N., Blackard, C., Boyles, C., Hassoin, B., Holmes, L. and Kreye, M. (1985). Marijuana: Prenatal and postnatal exposure in the human. In Pinkert, T.M. (ed.) *Current Research on the Consequences of Maternal Drug Abuse*, pp. 48–60. (NIDA Research Monograph 59, Washington, DC, Department of Health and Human Services)

6. Frank, D.A., Zuckerman, B.S., Amaro, H., Reece, H., Aboagye, K., Bauchner, H., Cabral, H., Fried, L., Hingson, R., Kayne, H., Levenson, S., Parker, S. and Vinci, R. Prevalence and correlates of cocaine use during pregnancy. *Pediatrics* (in press)

7. Kline, J., Stein, Z. and Hutzler, M. (1987). Cigarettes, alcohol and marijuana: Varying associations with birthweight. *Int. J. Epidemiol.*, **16**, 44–51

8. Hatch, E.E. and Bracken, M.B. (1986). Effect of marijuana use in pregnancy on fetal growth. *Am. J. Epidemiol.*, **124**, 986–993

9. Turner, C.E. (1980). Marijuana research and problems: an overview. *Pharm. Int.*, **1**, 93

10. Renault, P.F., Schuster, C.R., Heinrich, R. and Freeman, D.X. (1971). Marijuana: Standardized smoke administration and dose–effect curves on heart rate in humans. *Science*, **174**, 589

11. Kruez, D.S. and Axelrod, J. (1973). Delta-9-tetrahydrocannabinol: Localization in body fat. *Science*, **179**, 391

12. Nahar, G.G. (1976). *Marijuana: Chemistry, Biochemistry and Cellular Effects*. (New York: Springer-Verlag)

13. Smith, C.G. and Asch, R.H. Drug abuse and reproduction. *Fertil. Steril.*, **48**, 355–373

14. Mendelson, J.H. and Mello, N.K. (1984). Effects of marijuana on neuroendocrine hormones in human males and females. In *Marijuana Effects on the Endocrine and Reproductive Systems*. (NIDA Research Monograph, Washington, DC Government Printing Office)

15. Abel, E.L. (1984). *Smoking and Reproduction: An Annotated Bibliography*, pp. 11–12. (Boca Raton, FL: CRC Press)

16. Indanpaan-Haikkila, J. (1969). Placental transfer of titrated I tetrahydrocannabinol. *N. Engl. J. Med.*, **281**, 330

17. Abel, E.L. (1983). *Marijuana, Tobacco, Alcohol and Reproduction*. (Boca Raton, FL: CRC Press)

18. Abel, E.L. (1975). Cannabis: Effects on hunger and thirst. *Behav. Biol.*, **15**, 255

19. Abel, E.L. (1984). Effects of delta 9-THC on pregnancy and offspring in rats. *Neurobehav. Toxicol. Teratol.*, **6**, 29–32

20. Charlebois, A.J. and Fried, P.A. (1980). Interactive effects of nutrition and cannabis upon rat perinatal development. *Devel. Psychobiol.*, **13**, 591

21. Abel, E.L. (1985). Alcohol enhancement of marijuana-induced toxicity. *Teratology*, **31**, 35–40

22. Glatt, H., Ohlsson, A., Argurell, S. and Oesch, F. (1979). Delta-1-tetrahydrocannabinol and 1,2-epoxyhexahydrocannabinol: Mutagenicity investigation in the Ames test. *Mutat. Res.*, **66**, 329

23. Stenchever, M.A. and Allen, H. (1972). The effect of delta-9-tetrahydrocannabinol on the chromosomes of human lymphocytes in vitro. *Am. J. Obstet. Gynecol.*; **114**, 819

24. Greenland, S., Statish, D., Brown, N. and Gross, S.J. (1982). The effects of marijuana use during pregnancy. *Am. J. Obstet. Gynecol.*, **143**, 408

25. Tennes, M.A. and Blackard, C. (1980). Maternal alcohol consumption, birthweight and minor physical anomalies. *Am. J. Obstet. Gynecol.*, **138**, 774
26. O'Connell, C.M. and Fried, P.A. (1984). An investigation of prenatal cannabis exposure and minor physical anomalies in a low risk population. *Neurobehav. Toxicol. Teratol.*, **6**, 345
27. Amaro, H., Heeren, T., Morelock, S., Kayne, H., Hingson, R., Alpert, J.J. and Zuckerman, B. Maternal marijuana use and infant birth weight: Ethnic differences. (submitted for publication)
28. Hyser, Y., Anglin, M.D. and McGlothlin, W.H. (1987). Sex differences in addict careers: initiation of use. *Am. J. Drug Alcohol Abuse*, **13**, 33
29. Hingson, R., Zuckerman, B., Amaro, H., Frank, D., Kayne, H., Sorenson, J.R., Mitchell, J., Parker, S., Morelock, S. and Timperi, R. (1986). Maternal marijuana use and neonatal outcome: Uncertainty posed by self-reports. *Am. J. Public Health*, **76**, 667
30. Cone, E.J. and Johnson, R.E. (1986). Passive exposure to marijuana – subjective highs and objective urines. *Clin. Pharmacol. Ther.*, **40**, 247–56
31. Fried, P.A. (1980). Marijuana use by pregnant women: Neurobehavioral effects in neonates. *Drug Alcohol Depend.*, **6**, 415
32. Fried, P.A. and Makin, J.E. (1987). Neonatal behavioral correlates of prenatal exposure to marijuana, cigarettes and alcohol in a low risk population. *Neurobehav. Toxicol. Teratol.*, **9**, 1–7
33. Fried, P.A., Watkinson, B., Dillon, R.F. and Dulberg, C. (1987). Neonatal neurological status in a low-risk population after prenatal exposure to cigarettes, marijuana and alcohol. *J. Dev. Behav. Pediatr.*, **8**, 318–26
34. Simpson, W.J. (1975). A preliminary report of cigarette smoking and the incidence of prematurity. *Am. J. Obstet. Gynecol.*, **73**, 808
35. Fielding, J.E. (1978). Smoking and pregnancy. *N. Engl. J. Med.*, **298**, 337
36. US Public Health Service. (1979). *Smoking and Health*. A Report of the Surgeon General, US Department of Health, Education, and Welfare Publ. No. (PHS) 79-50066, Public Health Service, Office on Smoking and Health, Washington, DC
37. Quigley, M.E., Sheehan, K.L., Wilkes, M.M. and Yen, S.C.C. (1979). Effects of maternal smoking on circulatory catecholamine levels and fetal heart rates. *Am. J. Obstet. Gynecol.*, **133**, 685
38. Finnegan, L.P. (1985). Smoking and its effect on pregnancy and the newborn. In Harel, S. and Anaastasiow, N. (eds.) *The At-Risk Infant: Psycho/Socio/Medical Aspects.* pp. 127–136. (Baltimore, London: Paul H. Brookes Publishing Co., Inc.)
39. Kline, J., Stein, Z.A. and Susser, M. (1977). Smoking as a risk factor for spontaneous abortion. *N. Engl. J. Med.*, **297**, 793
40. Himmelberger, D.U., Brown, B.W. and Cohen, E.N. (1978). Cigarette smoking during pregnancy and the occurrence of spontaneous abortion and congenital abnormality. *Am. J. Epidemiol.*, **108**, 470
41. Bergman, A.B. and Wiesner, L.A. (1976). Relationship of passive cigarette smoking to sudden infant death syndrome. *Pediatrics*, **58**, 665
42. Lewak, N., Van-den-Berg, B.J. and Beckwith, J.B. (1979). Sudden infant death syndrome risk factors: Prospective data review. *Clin. Pediatr.*, **18**, 404
43. Naeye, R.L., Ladis, B. and Drage, J.S. (1976). Sudden infant death syndrome. *Am. J. Dis. Child.*, **130**, 1207
44. O'Lane, J.M. (1963). Some fetal effects of maternal cigarette smoking. *Obstet. Gynecol.*, **22**, 181
45. Garn, S.M., Johnson, M., Ridella, S.A. and Zetzold, A.S. (1981). Effects of maternal cigarette smoking on Apgar scores. *Am. J. Dis. Child.*, **135**, 503
46. Schramm, W. (1980). Smoking and pregnancy outcome. *Mod. Med.*, **77**, 619
47. Hingson, R., Gould, J.R., Morelock, S., Kayne, H., Heeren, T., Alpert, J.J., Zuckerman, B. and Day, N. (1982). Maternal cigarette smoking, psychoactive substance use and infant Apgar scores. *Am. J. Obstet. Gynecol.*, **144**, 959
48. Haddow, J.E., Knight, G.J., Palomaki, G.E., Kloza, E.M. and Wald, N.J. (1987). Cigarette consumption and serum cotinine in relation to birthweight. *Br. J. Obstet. Gynaecol.*, **94**, 678

49. Sexton, M. and Hebel, J.R. (1984). A clinical trial of change in maternal smoking and its effect on birth weight. *J. Am. Med. Assoc.*, **251**, 911

50. Harrison, G.G., Branson, R.S. and Vaugher, Y.E. (1983). Association of maternal smoking with body composition of the newborn. *Am. J. Clin. Nutr.*, **38**, 757

51. Miller, H.C., Hassanein, K. and Hensleigh, P. (1976). Fetal growth retardation in relation to maternal smoking and weight gain in pregnancy. *Am. J. Obstet. Gynecol.*, **1**, 55

52. Davies, D.P., Gray, O.P., Ellwood, P.C. and Abernethy, M. (1976). Cigarette smoking in pregnancy: Associations with maternal weight gain and fetal growth. *Lancet*, **1**, 385

53. Fedick, J., Alberman, E. and Goldstein, H. (1971). Possible teratogenic effect of cigarette smoking. *Nature (London)*, **231**, 530

54. Heinonen, O.P. (1976). Risk factors for congenital heart disease: A prospective study. In Kelly, S., Hook, E.B. and Janerich, D.T. (eds.) *Birth Defects Risks and Consequences*, pp. 221–264. (New York: Academic Press)

55. Andrews, J. and McGarry, J.M. (1972). A community study of smoking in pregnancy. *J. Obstet. Gynaecol. Br. Commonw.*, **79**, 1057

56. Peterson, W.F., Morese, K.N. and Kaltreider, D.F. (1965). Smoking and prematurity: A preliminary report based on study of 7740 caucasians. *Obstet. Gynecol.*, **26**, 775

57. Kullander, S. and Kallan, B. (1971). A prospective study of smoking and pregnancy. *Acta Obstet. Gynaecol. Scand.*, **50**, 83

58. Richards, I.D. (1969). Congenital malformations and environmental influences in pregnancy. *Br. J. Prev. Soc. Med.*, **23**, 218

59. Saxton, D.W. (1978). The behaviour of infants whose mothers smoke in pregnancy. *Early Hum. Devel.*, **2**, 363

60. Martin, J.C., Martin, D.C. and Lund, C. (1973). Maternal alcohol ingestion and cigarette smoking and their effect upon newborn conditioning. *Alcohol Clin. Exp. Res.*, **1**, 243

61. Landesman-Dwyer, S., Keller, L.S. and Streissguth, A.P. (1978). Naturalistic observations of newborns: Effects of maternal alcohol intake. *Alcohol Clin. Exp. Res.*, **2**, 171

62. Woodson, E.M., DaCosta, P. and Woodson, R.H. (1980). Maternal smoking and newborn behavior. Presented at the *International Conference on Infant Studies*, New Haven, CT

63. Picone, T.A., Allen, L.H., Olsen, P.N. and Ferris, M.E. (1982). Pregnancy outcome in North American Women. II Effects of diet, cigarette smoking, stress, and weight gain on placentas, and on neonatal physical and behavioral characteristics. *Am. J. Clin. Nutr.*, **36**, 1214

64. Butler, N.R. and Goldstein, H. (1973). Smoking in pregnancy and subsequent child development. *Br. Med. J.*, **4**, 573

65. Dunn, H.G., McBurney, A.K., Ingram, S. and Hunter, C.M. (1977). Maternal cigarette smoking during pregnancy and the child's subsequent development. II. Neurological and intellectual maturation to the age of 6.5 years. *Can. J. Publ. Health*, **68**, 43

6

Cocaine: The Drug of Choice

William T Atkins

The drug of choice for many drug-dependent pregnant women, cocaine, is also one of the most powerfully addicting substances of human abuse. Cocaine use in America has increased dramatically in the past few years and has become a severe health problem for all of our citizens. It has gone from a potion that was utilized only by South American Indians to a multibillion dollar illegal industry. Cocaine has quickly become the drug of choice for millions of Americans because of its 'Hollywood' image, coupled with its euphoric effects and the more effective marketing practices used by dealers. According to the latest National Institute on Drug Abuse Household Drug Survey[1], cocaine is the only drug that has shown a constant increase in the number of users in the 1980s. The number of people trying cocaine at least once has increased from 5.4 million in 1974 to almost 23 million in 1985. This increase in use has also meant increases in emergency room cases associated with cocaine, rising treatment admissions for cocaine problems and increasing cocaine-induced deaths[2].

Cocaine can no longer be thought of as a drug with no addicting properties. The reinforcing nature of cocaine, coupled with more intensified use and more effective delivery systems, leads many users to a pattern of compulsive use which ultimately can cause disruption in families, problems in job performance as well as physical and mental deterioration, if not death.

The epidemic proportions of cocaine use and its increased use is attributable to increases in supply, decreases in cost and increased addictive potential, and, although the prevalence of cocaine usage now may be stabilizing, the intensity of usage has increased with intravenous and freebase self-administration.

A closer look at the national figures reveals that since the early 1970s, the incidence of cocaine use has been increasing to astronomic proportions[1,3-5]. The percentage of youth between the ages of 12-17 using cocaine within the past year has risen from 1.5 in 1972 to 4.4 in 1985. Among young adults, 18-25, use within the past year has risen from 8.1% in 1974 to 16.4% in 1985. Among the adult population, those over age 26, the yearly use of cocaine increased from 0.6% in 1976 to 4.2% in 1985. Current use, defined as use in the past month, is also increasing for all age groups. The youth population shows current use increasing from 0.6% in 1972 to 1.8% in 1985. This is an estimated 518,000 current users in this age group. For the young adult age group, current use has gone from 3.1% in 1974 to 7.7% in 1985, or 3,056,000 current users, and, for the adult population, current use went from negligible amounts to 2% in 1985, or 5,700,000 current users.

The users of cocaine, as well as other illicit drugs, are still predominantly male. However, the gap between male and female users appears to be narrowing. The 1985 NIDA Household Survey indicated that, among adults age 18–44, approximately two-thirds of those who had ever used cocaine were male, as were almost 70% of the current users. In contrast, among youth age 12–17, approximately 50% were male, indicating a trend toward increasing use among females. Data from the High School Survey suggests a similar pattern, with 42% of current users of cocaine being female[3]. The implications of this increased use of cocaine by women will mean more obstetrical problems for those who become pregnant.

A closer analysis of these data provides some important information pertaining to future trends. The data show the young adult population, age 18–25, as the predominant cocaine-using group. Since 1979, however, the use by youth and the young adult population continues to escalate. Edgar Adams and his associates[5] have suggested that this increase in cocaine use among older adults is a cohort effect: that is, the result of the aging of the adult population rather than the result of new use in the older population. Their findings indicate that the significant increases in the number of lifetime and annual cocaine users were only partially explained by a cohort effect. Thus, not only is there a high number of young adults using cocaine, but a significant number from this age group will begin using cocaine after age 26. This suggests that the period of risk for cocaine use increases steadily after age 20 and lasts longer than that for other drugs. In women, these dates coincide with the child-bearing age range, setting the stage for an escalation in cocaine-induced prenatal complications.

CRACK AND FREEBASING

A primary concern for the drug treatment field is the marketing of a new form of cocaine called crack. Named for the crackling sound the powder makes when heated and vaporized into smoke inside small glass containers, crack can elevate the purity of 'street' cocaine from 20–30% to as much as 80%. 'Street' cocaine varies greatly in purity, generally depending upon the quantity of the purchase. Kilogram and pound purchases are usually 90%

pure, ounces are often 70–80% pure, and grams may vary from 10–80% pure cocaine. Crack is 10 to 20 times more potent than powdered street cocaine and reaches the brain in less than 30 seconds. People who snort cocaine become addicted after an average **four years** of use, but heavy crack users can become addicted within **two weeks**[6]. Of the 6 to 10 million regular cocaine users in the nation, as many as 1 to 2 million have turned to crack in the last 18 months[7].

The phenomenon of crack use differs from previous cocaine use patterns in two ways: (1) in the past, the user made the conversion from cocaine hydrochloride to freebase; today the product is being sold as freebase and (2) the introduction of a unit dose concept to the drug market effectively removes the initial price barrier in that population where price previously precluded experimentation. Because of its highly addictive nature, crack users buy more of the substance, and it thus becomes more expensive than cocaine hydrochloride.

Freebasing or smoking cocaine as a route of administration has increased from less than 1% in 1977 to almost 5% in 1981 and 18% in 1984[1,6]. Thus, smoking or freebasing as a route of administration was gaining in popularity prior to the introduction of crack. However, the availability of crack or freebase may have served to accelerate this trend. In a population admitted to the Chemical Dependence Program of Northwestern Memorial Hospital, the route of administration most often reported (43.9%) was freebasing[8,9]. The patients who used the largest quantities of cocaine at each episode were smoking cocaine freebase. In a study at Yale, cocaine freebase users smoked twice as much cocaine weekly as i.v. users or snorters consumed and used almost twice as much per run as did the rest of the sample[6].

ADVERSE CONSEQUENCES OF COCAINE USE

The increased use of cocaine has had a drastic impact on the number of reported emergency room cases and deaths related to this drug[2]. Between 1981 and 1985, the number of hospital emergencies associated with the use of cocaine increased threefold, from 3,296 to 9,946. Over the two most recent years, the number of cocaine-related hospital emergencies increased 17%, from 8,470 to 9,946.

In 1977, emergency room data reflected that less than 1% of cases were associated with smoking cocaine. By 1984, 6% of emergency room cases were associated with smoking. Preliminary data for the first quarter of 1986 indicated that 14.3% of all cocaine cases reported smoking as the route of administration. In 1985, smoking cocaine represented 11% of all mentions. The primary cities involved were Los Angeles, 34.5% of mentions, Chicago,

10.3% of mentions and New York, 4.3% of all mentions.

Between 1981 and 1984, the number of cocaine-related deaths increased almost threefold, from 195 to 580. Provisional data for 1985 indicates that cocaine-related deaths are continuing at unprecedented high levels, with 563 deaths reported to date. Morbidity data from the nation's largest city, New York, are not included in these statistics.

COCAINE IN ILLINOIS

Cocaine addiction is also still on the upswing in Illinois. This drug continues to be the only drug with a steady rise in treatment admissions to the publicly funded treatment programs. Cocaine-abuse treatment admissions represent 18% of the 1985 Department of Alcoholism and Substance Abuse admissions. This is compared to only 12% in 1984. Among this 1986 treatment group, males are still disproportionately represented, 70.5% to 29.5% females. There are 56.3% whites admitted, 39.4% blacks, 4.1% Latinos and 0.3% others[10]. These figures are not fully reflective of the extent of the cocaine problem. The client admissions data to state-supported drug abuse programs do not inclulde private and hospital-based program admissions. Data collected from some of these treatment centers show that the clientele at these private treatment centers are more likely to be younger, employed, high-income individuals with health insurance than those in the state-funded programs. These private programs also report a higher proportion of cocaine abusers seeking treatment.

Further underscoring the extent of cocaine-related problems in Illinois is the fact that since 1984 cocaine has continually surpassed all other single substances in contributing to emergency room episodes in Chicago as reported by DAWN (Drug Abuse Warning Network)[2]. Previously, heroin/morphine and diazepam significantly outranked cocaine in leading to adverse reactions requiring emergency room treatment. Acute reactions to cocaine have contributed to an increase from 47 first quarter cocaine mentions in 1983 to 239 first quarter mentions in 1986. The percentage of these mentions in Chicago administered by smoking has increased from 2.1% in the first quarter of 1983 to 10% in the first quarter of 1986. This route of administration has been shown to cause more severe addictions and has greater health consequences.

This steady climb of cocaine usage by the citizens of Illinois and the United States presents numerous problems for policymakers, administrators and treatment staff in the alcoholism and substance-abuse treatment field. There is a primary need to steadily increase treatment capacity throughout the country to meet the needs of the growing population seeking treatment[11].

This task is made more difficult by the fact that many states are in a time of tight fiscal spending.

Secondly, the changing demographics of cocaine abusers show that the number of women, youth and minorities seeking treatment is increasing so that further refinement and broadening of the treatment base to better meet the needs of these special population groups will be necessary. For example, cocaine dependency among women of child-bearing age (18–34) continues to increase. Due to the adverse consequences for the mother and infant, this high-risk population must be targeted for increased intervention, prevention and treatment contact within the field. The field must develop the skills and knowledge needed to identify these individuals and the capability to properly refer and counsel these women.

A third major issue is the growing evidence that cocaine appears to be different from other drugs in its addiction potential. Thus, individual states and programs may have to re-examine and perhaps modify their treatment regimens to adequately serve the needs of cocaine addicts.

The treatment of cocaine dependency must begin with a thorough assessment of the extent of cocaine use. Quantity, frequency, duration and mode of administration must be determined. Progression of use, from intranasal to smoking, is important, as is a detailed history of concomitant drug use. Polydrug abuse is common, with only 10–30% of abusers admitted to hospital treatment programs reporting abuse of only cocaine[12]. Although some multiple abusers have a long history of abuse of other drugs prior to their involvement with cocaine, others have been only recreational users of alcohol or marijuana and are taken by surprise by their addiction, because cocaine is the first drug they have 'lost control over'. Treatment centers must be sensitized to the extent of the multidrug user problem. Proper treatment must deal with all possible addiction problems.

Treatment of crack and cocaine addiction is increasingly becoming a controversial topic in the drug-abuse treatment field. Traditionally, drug addiction has been viewed as a psychosocial disease that can be curbed only through discipline and abstinence, both of which need to be reinforced by group therapy. However, recent evidence shows that cocaine produces euphoric effects by manipulating the chemistry of the brain, and a pharmacological agent that will block or reverse this manipulation may be needed[12]. The magnitude of the cocaine-abuse epidemic makes it imperative for the field to conduct further research into the applicability of these pharmacologic inhibitors. This information should be disseminated along with a unified national stance on the issue.

Irrespective of pharmacological interventions, psychological approaches at present remain the most successful aspect of treatment for cocaine addiction[8,9,13]. An optimal treatment plan must include therapy with participation in a cocaine recovery group. Group sessions have been successful because they provide positive role models, a ready-made peer support network and an excellent form for discussing a wide range of issues that are crucial to abstinence and recovery. Individual therapy sessions complement the group meetings but should focus more on personal and psychodynamic issues pertaining to relationships, sexual functioning, self-esteem, family problems and other issues underlying the drug use. This entire process is long and arduous and fraught with a high relapse rate. An estimated 75% of cocaine addicts seeking treatment for the first time fail to achieve abstinence[8,9].

Information about the dangers of cocaine abuse are beginning to be understood by the public through public education campaigns. Although prevalence estimates on the cocaine problem may have peaked, as some have suggested, treatment figures show that more and more people are seeking help for cocaine abuse, among them pregnant women. The threat posed to the infants of these pregnant women heightens the need for preventive efforts directed at this population.

REFERENCES

1. National Institute of Drug Abuse. *Drug Abuse Indicator Trends.* Community Epidemiology Work Group Proceedings, Vol.1, June 1986
2. Colliver, J. (1986). *A Decade of DAWN: Cocaine Related Cases, 1976–85.* (Rockville, MD: NIDA)
3. Johnston, L. *et al.* (1986). *Highlights from Drugs and American High School Students 1975–1985.* (Rockville, MD: NIDA)
4. Johnston, L. *et al.* (1984). *Highlights from Drugs and American High School Students 1975–1983.* (Rockville, MD: NIDA)
5. Adams, E. *et al.* (1987). *Trends in Prevalence and Consequences of Cocaine Use.* (Washington, DC: Haworth Press)
6. Weiss, R. *et al.* (1986). Subtypes of cocaine abuse. *Psychiatr. Clin. N. Am.,* 9, 3–10
7. Issacs, S. *et al.* (1987). Crack abuse: a problem of the eighties. *Oral Surg.,* 63, 12–16
8. Schick, J.F. and Senay, E. (1986). *Directions in Psychiatry.* Part 1
9. Schick, J.F. and Senay, E. (1986). *Directions in Psychiatry.* Part 2
10. Gross, J. (1985). *Cocaine in Illinois.* (Chicago. IL: Illinois Department of Alcoholism and Substance Abuse)
11. Illinois Department of Alcoholism and Substance Abuse (1987). Comprehensive state plan for alcoholism and substance abuse services. FY86–FY88
12. Adler, M. *et al.* (1987). Scientific perspectives on cocaine abuse. *Pharmacology,* 29, 20–27
13. O'Connell, K. (April 1986). A behavioral treatment approach to the treatment of cocaine addiction. *Proceedings of the International Congress on Drug Prevention and Treatment,* NIDA, Rockville, MD

7

Cocaine: Effects on Pregnancy and the Neonate

Ira J Chasnoff

With the increased use of cocaine in the United States, it has been recently recognized that increasing numbers of pregnancies are complicated by cocaine use[1]. Information regarding the effects of cocaine on the devloping fetus and newborn infant is sparse, however, and thus far has focused on cocaine users as a group. There has been no information regarding the relationship of patterns of cocaine use in pregnancy and differential effects on outcome of pregnancy or the newborn infant. In the present chapter, pregnancies complicated by the abuse of cocaine are presented and compared to pregnancies in which no alcohol and/or drug use occurred. These cocaine-exposed pregnancies are then evaluated according to patterns of cocaine use in the pregnancy.

COCAINE AND PREGNANCY

From January, 1976 to July, 1987, 75 infants were born to cocaine-using women enrolled in the Perinatal Center for Chemical Dependence. Each of these women used cocaine intranasally, intravenously or by freebasing in the first trimester of pregnancy, and 45 (60%) of the women continued to use cocaine throughout the pregnancy. Urine samples were obtained on a regular basis to screen for the use of licit and illicit drugs (opiates, amphetamines, barbiturates, marijuana, benzodiazepines, propoxyphene, cocaine, phencyclidine, tobacco and alcohol).

A drug-free comparison group ($n = 70$) was selected from the population of the Prentice Ambulatory Care Clinic representing women of a similar racial and socioeconomic distribution. These women had no history or evidence of licit or illicit drug use and were selected for the control group on the basis of social, demographic and environmental backgrounds as well as being comparable for cigarette use during pregnancy (Table 7.1). Management of pregnancy was similar for the two groups of women and has been described in previous publications[2,3].

Table 7.1 Maternal characteristics*

	Cocaine	Drug-free
n	70	70
	X	X
Age (years)	26.7	27.1
Gravidity	3.5	2.7
Cigarettes/day	12.7	9.2
Alcohol (cc/week)	16.7 (7 women)	–
Marijuana (joints/month)	7.8	–
Weight gain (pounds)	27.1	28.6
Education (years)	11.4	11.0

* t-test, not significant

Table 2 Complications of labor and delivery*

	Cocaine		Drug-free	
	n	%	n	%
Premature labor	18	24	2	3.0
Precipitous labor	7	9	2	3.0
Abruptio placentae	12	16	1	1.0
Fetal monitor abnormality	7	9	4	5.0

* chi^2 analysis, $p < 0.05$ for all results

Table 3 Neonatal growth parameters*

	Cocaine X	Drug-free X
Weight (g)	3094	3473
Length (cm)	48.9	51.1
Head circumference (cm)	33.1	34.8

* t-test, $p < 0.05$

The reproductive histories of all women were reviewed, and labor and delivery data recorded at the time of delivery. All neonates were examined at birth. As in other substance-abusing populations, the cocaine-addicted

98

women had a high incidence of infectious disease complications, especially hepatitis (24%) and venereal disease (10.5%). There was an increase in complications of labor and delivery in cocaine-using women as compared to drug-free women (Table 7.2) and an increased incidence of premature labor.

All the infants were of singleton birth, and there was a similar distribution of infants according to sex in each group. A similar number of infants in each group had Apgar scores less than 7 at one and five minutes. Meconium staining occurred in the cocaine-exposed group with greater frequency as compared to the control group of infants. Mean gestational age was reduced for the cocaine group of infants (37.1 *vs.* 39.3 weeks). Eliminating premature infants, there was a statistically significant difference in birth weights, lengths and head circumference between infants in the two groups (Table 7.3).

The perinatal complications with the greatest implications for long-term prognoses for the cocaine-exposed infants were the reduced mean gestational age and the high rate (19%) of small-for-gestational age neonates in the cocaine group as compared to 3% of infants in the control group (3% SGA).

No infant in the cocaine group required pharmacologic therapy for symptoms of abstinence. Nine cocaine-exposed infants had malformations of the genitourinary tract: two with 'prune belly syndrome', one with female pseudohermaphroditism, three with a first or second degree hypospadias and undescended testis, and three with hydronephrosis. Two infants in the cocaine group suffered a perinatal cerebral infarction related to their mother's cocaine use in the 48 to 72 hours prior to delivery.

The majority of the cocaine-exposed infants could be classified as 'fragile' infants with very low thresholds for overstimulation. These infants required a great deal of assistance from caretakers to maintain control of their hyperexcitable nervous systems. This fragility of the cocaine-exposed infants is seen clearly in their responses on the Brazelton Neonatal Behavioral Assessment Scale[4] and is discussed in a later chapter.

PATTERNS OF COCAINE USE

A second analysis of outcome of cocaine-exposed pregnancies was performed in February, 1988. From January 1, 1986 to December 31, 1987, 108 women who had used cocaine during their pregnancies received prenatal care at the Perinatal Center for Chemical Dependence. All women were enrolled by the 25th week of pregnancy and received intensive obstetric care. The goal of psychotherapeutic intervention was to bring the women to abstinence. Urine toxicology through EMIT screening was performed at admission with positive results confirmed by GC/MS. At each prenatal obstetric visit, current substance abuse history was reviewed and additional urines for toxicology were regularly obtained. History and toxicology studies covered the substances previously noted. At time of delivery, cocaine-using women were divided into two groups. The first group (Group I) consisted of 35 women who conceived on cocaine, but who reached abstinence by the end of the second trimester and had no further cocaine use throughout their pregnancy. The second group of cocaine-using women (Group II) consisted of 73 women who conceived on cocaine and, despite being enrolled in the comprehensive program, continued to use cocaine throughout their pregnancy.

The two groups of patients were similar for maternal age, gravidity, prenatal weight gain, and racial distribution. Drug use patterns for the two cocaine groups were also similar (i.e. cocaine use amount, frequency, and route of administration and alcohol and marijuana use). Use of tobacco cigarettes throughout pregnancy was also similar for both groups.

Perinatal outcome is summarized in Table 7.4. Infants born to women who used cocaine throughout pregnancy had a lower mean gestational age than infants in the other group. Infants born to women who used cocaine only in the first trimester had a mean gestation at full term. The incidence of intrauterine growth retardation and premature births were also increased in the third trimester-exposed pregnancies. Interestingly, use of cocaine in only the first trimester was associated with an increased rate of abruptio placentae as compared to the general population, similar to infants born to mothers who used cocaine throughout pregnancy.

Table 7.4 Perinatal complications: patterns of cocaine use

	Cocaine: 2 trimester	*Cocaine: 3 trimester*
n	35	73
Gestation age (X)	38.3	37
SGA*	2%	20%
Premature delivery**	3%	24%
Abruptio placentae	8%	13%

* Small-for-gestational age
** <38 weeks gestation

Evaluation of neonatal growth parameters showed that full-term infants born to mothers who used cocaine throughout pregnancy had a lower mean weight, length, and head circumference at birth when compared to the first two trimesters-exposed full-term infants (Table 7.5).

Table 7.5 Neonatal growth parameters: patterns of cocaine use

	Cocaine: 2 trimester	Cocaine: 3 trimester
n^*	34	56
	X	X
Weight (g)	3211	2812
Length (cm)	49	47.6
Head circumference (cm)	33.5	32.5

* Infants > 38 weeks gestation

IMPLICATIONS FOR HEALTH CARE DELIVERY

Current studies have shown that a significant number of women in the child-bearing range 18–35 years of age are actively using cocaine[5]. Many of these women become pregnant and continue to use cocaine without realizing that they are pregnant. Thus, it is important to evaluate the effects of cocaine use in early pregnancy rather than its effects only when used throughout pregnancy. In addition, development of intervention programs for cocaine-using pregnant women will necessarily rely on information regarding the possibility of improved outcome for pregnancies in which a woman stops using cocaine in the first trimester of pregnancy.

In the present study, it was found that cessation of cocaine use by the end of the second trimester improved obstetric outcome. An increased proportion of pregnancies were able to go to full term and there was an improvement in intrauterine growth if the mother stopped using cocaine in the early part of pregnancy. Surprisingly, the rate of abruptio placentae did not decrease if a woman abstained from cocaine in the last trimester of pregnancy. It has been hypothesized that the high rate of abruptio placentae in cocaine-exposed pregnancies is related to the acute hypertension produced by cocaine use[1]. However, in the present study it appears that the damage done to placental and uterine vessels in early pregnancy by the cocaine places these pregnancies at continued risk even if cocaine use ceases.

Recent studies have confirmed that maternal cocaine use is related to intrauterine growth retardation[6]. In the present study, infants exposed to cocaine throughout pregnancy had a decrease in mean birth weight, length and head circumference compared to the infants exposed in the first two trimesters. It has been hypothesized that this decrease in intrauterine growth is related to the intermittent diminution of placental blood flow associated

101

with maternal cocaine use. Infants whose mothers used cocaine in the first two trimesters had improved intrauterine growth. Thus, although the effect of alcohol, marijuana and tobacco use and the interaction of these agents with cocaine cannot be completely evaluated at this point, it appears that cocaine use was a major factor in the growth impairment, since the infants exposed to cocaine in only the first two trimesters were exposed to similar amounts of alcohol, marijuana and tobacco as the second group of infants.

A recent study completed at the Perinatal Center for Chemical Dependence demonstrated genitourinary tract malformations in infants exposed to cocaine in pregnancy[7]. Other malformations, including CNS, have been reported for cocaine-exposed infants. In addition, three infants in our population have had ileal atresia. A recent paper attributes neural tube defects to a fetal vascular basis[9]. This theory coincides with cocaine's pharmacologic effects of vasoconstriction, including marked vasoconstriction for placental and fetal vessels[10].

Two infants whose mothers used cocaine in the two days prior to delivery suffered cerebral infarctions which were thought to have occurred in the perinatal period. The cardiovascular effects of cocaine have been well documented and increasing numbers of young adults who use cocaine have developed myocardial infarctions and cerebral infarctions[11].

Apnea of infancy whereby infants suffered a period of apnea, paleness and/or cyanosis occurred in nine of the cocaine-exposed infants with no correlation between incidence and pattern of cocaine exposure. Recent work has established the increased risk of sudden infant death syndrome in infants exposed to various substances of abuse, especially cocaine[12], and the question remains as to the significance of apnea in this special population.

Little reliable information regarding long-term outcome of infants passively exposed to cocaine is available. To best evaluate these children at school age, environmental factors must be taken into account. These environmental factors are not only socioeconomic but should encompass aspects of the mother–infant relationship, including psychopathology and personality. Further studies are needed before final conclusions can be drawn as to the long-term effects of *in utero* drug exposure on infant and child development.

The developmental risks imposed by the maternal use of cocaine are, perhaps, more than many other risk factors, preventable. However, prevention of the problem requires education of the public and professional sectors. Few individuals, including primary care physicians, recognize the hazards that cocaine presents to the pregnant woman and her unborn child. Until these hazards do become general knowledge, the increasing numbers of pregnant women using cocaine will continue to rise. Appropriate intervention for women who are using cocaine when they become pregnant must rely on comprehensive history taking and examination by health care professionals. Evidence for improved outcome related to cessation of cocaine in early pregnancy is now available. The pharmacologic characteristics of cocaine support this clinical information. Further research into this area must focus not only on the effects of cocaine *per se*, but also the interactive effects of polydrug use, the dynamics of maternal/infant interaction in a substance-abusing mother, and environmental factors which place these infants at high risk for future medical and developmental disabilities.

REFERENCES

1. Chasnoff, I.J., Burns, W.J., Schnoll, S.H. and Burns, K.A. (1985). Cocaine use in pregnancy. *N. Engl. J. Med.*, **313**, 666
2. Chasnoff, I.J. (1985). Effects of maternal narcotic vs. non-narcotic addiction on neonatal neurobehavior and infant development. In Pinkert, T.M. (ed.) *Consequences of Maternal Drug Abuse*, pp. 84–95. (Washington, DC: National Institute on Drug Abuse)
3. Chasnoff, I.J., Hatcher, R. and Burns, W.J. (1982). Polydrug- and methadone-addicted newborns. A continuum of impairment? *Pediatrics*, **70**, 210
4. Brazelton, T.B. (1968). *Neonatal Behavioral Assessment Scale*. (Philadelphia: Spastics International)
5. Abelson, H.I. and Miller, J.D. (1985). A decade of trends in cocaine use in the household population. *Natl. Inst. Drug Abuse Res. Monogr. Ser.*, **61**, 35
6. NacGregor, S.N., Keith, L.G., Chasnoff, I.J., Rosner, M.A., Chisum, G.M., Shaw, P. and Minogue, J.P. (1987). Cocaine use during pregnancy: adverse perinatal outcome. *Am. J. Obstet. Gynecol.*, **157**, 686
7. Chasnoff, I.J., Chisum, G.M. and Kaplan, W. (1988). Maternal cocaine use and genitourinary tract malformations. *Teratology*, **37**, 201
8. Bingol, N., Fuchs, M., Diaz, V., Stone, R.K. and Gromisch, D.S. (1987). Teratogenicity of cocaine in humans. *J. Pediatr.*, **110**, 93
9. Stevenson, R.E., Kelly, J.C., Aylsworth, A.S. and Phelan, M.C. (1987). Vascular basis for neural tube defects: a hypothesis. *Pediatrics*, **80**, 102
10. Ritchie, J.M. and Greene, N.M. (1980). Local anesthesia. In Gilman, A.G., Goodman, L.S. and Gilman, A. (eds.) *The Pharmacological Basis of Therapeutics*, pp. 300–320. (New York: Macmillan)
11. Cregler, L. and Mark, H. (1986). Medical complications of cocaine abuse. *N. Engl. J. Med.*, **315**, 1495
12. Ward, S.L., Schutz, S. and Kirshna, V. (1986). Abnormal sleeping ventilatory patterns in infants of substance-abusing mothers. *Am. J. Dis. Child.*, **140**, 1015

8

The Effects of Perinatal Cocaine Exposure on Infant Neurobehavior and Early Maternal – Infant Interactions

Dan R Griffith

INTRODUCTION

Researchers exploring the nature of maternal – infant relationships have paid increasing attention in recent years to the roles of both mother and infant in determining the quantity and quality of mother – infant interactions[1-8]. Infants enter into the maternal – infant relationship with individual temperaments, specific needs, and varying capabilities to organize their environments. Mothers begin the relationship with their own individual expectations about their infants, capacities for recognizing and responding to their infant's needs, and needs of their own.

In order to build an optimally functioning maternal – infant relationship which is fulfilling to both partners, mother and infant must each have the behavioral repertoire and the adaptability to respond appropriately to the stimulation provided by the other. If the infant has difficulty responding to environmental demands in an organized fashion, then it is the responsibility of the mother to sustain the mother – infant relationship by modulating her stimulation to fit the information-processing needs of the infant[3]. When the mother is unable to fulfill this function, the infant is likely to be exposed repeatedly to experiences which overwhelm him/her and impede rather than facilitate his/her development[8].

In our work with women who abused cocaine during pregnancy and with their infants at the Perinatal Center for Chemical Dependency of Northwestern University, we have seen this type of non-functional, often detrimental maternal – infant relationship all too frequently. In the following pages, I will describe the response deficits we have observed in cocaine-exposed infants, some of the problems common to drug-abusing women which might interfere with their maternal effectiveness, and our beginning efforts to teach the mothers in our program how to provide adequate stimulation for their infants.

THE COCAINE-EXPOSED INFANTS

The infants to be discussed here were full-term infants born to women who abused cocaine with or without other drugs at some time during their pregnancy. The vast majority of these infants can be classified as fragile infants who have very low thresholds for overstimulation and require a great deal of assistance from caretakers to maintain control of their hyperexcitable nervous systems. This fragility of the cocaine-exposed infant is seen clearly in their responses to many of the items on the Neonatal Behavioral Assessment Scale (NBAS)[9]. Infants in our program are assessed with the NBAS between 16 hours and 3 days of life (the newborn period), at 1 week of age, and at 1 month of age. Throughout the first month of life, these infants as a group had difficulties responding appropriately to the demands of testing. It is important to note, however, that there was considerable variability from infant to infant with regard to both the severity of the initial response deficiencies and the rate of recovery.

State Control in the Cocaine-Exposed Infant

Ongoing research confirms data from an earlier study[10] which indicated that newborn cocaine-exposed infants had the most difficulty functioning in the areas of state control and orientation. The state control dimension refers to the infant's ability to move appropriately through the various states of arousal in response to the demands of the environment. During NBAS testing, the well-organized, fully functioning infant will move through each of the states of arousal, including sleep states, a drowsy state, an alert responsive state, an agitated state, and a crying state. Each state achieved will be appropriate for the level and type of stimulation the infant is encountering, and the transition from state to state will be relatively smooth. The newborn cocaine-exposed infants, however, are almost never well-organized, fully functioning infants. Instead they spend most of their time in states which shut them off from external stimulation, and their state changes tend to be abrupt and inappropriate for the level of stimulation encountered.

During NBAS testing of cocaine-exposed newborns, we have observed four common patterns of state control. In the first pattern, the infants pull down into a deep sleep in response to the first stimulation received and remain asleep throughout the exam. They do not awaken even though they might be undressed, rocked, talked to, and physically manipulated. In fact, infants displaying this pattern seem to pull into a deeper sleep the more we try to wake them up. If they awaken at all, it is only after we have swaddled them and placed them in their bassinets in quiet, darkened rooms. Under

's conditions many of the infants will begin to open their
___nd. They will, however, shut down again as soon as we try
___m, whether it be through auditory, visual, or tactile stimulation.
___, if the infants are aware that deep sleep is their only and best
___ against being over-stimulated and losing control of themselves.

The second pattern of state control demonstrated by newborn cocaine-exposed infants is similar to the first in that the infant cannot or will not wake up during the course of the entire NBAS exam. They appear to be worse off than the first group, however, because they cannot seem to pull into a deep enough sleep to avoid stimulation. Throughout the exam, they startle, whimper, change colors, breath irregularly, and thrash about, in response to the stimuli presented, yet, they never awaken. These infants seem unable to either attend to or shut-out external stimulation.

Newborn cocaine-exposed infants displaying the third pattern of state control vacillate between sleep states and cry states throughout the exam. Their response to most tactile stimulation and sometimes auditory stimulation is to move abruptly from sleeping to agitated crying. As soon as the stimulation is terminated, they pull down into their sleep shelter again. Some of these infants require tight swaddling to maintain their sleep state. As soon as they are unwrapped, they change color, begin thrashing their arms about, and quickly escalate to uncontrolled crying until they are swaddled again. Once reswaddled, they return to sleep. The infants displaying this pattern do not achieve any attention to or responsiveness to visual or auditory stimuli during the NBAS exam.

The final and most common pattern of state control for newborn cocaine-exposed infants is similar to the third pattern in that these infants tend to use both sleeping and crying to shut themselves off from excessive stimulation. These infants, however, if managed carefully by the examiner, are able to reach very brief periods of alert responsiveness. The quality of these alert periods and the types of examiner facilitation frequently needed to achieve them will be described in detail later in this chapter.

By the time the cocaine-exposed infants have reached one month of age, their state control abilities as measured by the NBAS have improved but are still significantly below those of drug-free newborns[11]. Most of the one-month-old cocaine-exposed infants are capable of reaching all of the various states of arousal including brief periods of alert responsiveness. Many of them, however, still have very low thresholds for overstimulation and require a great deal of careful handling and containment from the examiner in order to reach and/or maintain responsive states. Without examiner assistance, they often display abrupt, inappropriate state changes in response to the demands of the exam. Even with the organizational assistance provided by the examiner, there are a few one-month-old cocaine-exposed infants who seem unable to tolerate even low levels of stimulation. These infants quickly achieve an agitated cry state in response to most types of stimulation. These cry states are long-lasting and seemingly self-perpetuating. The crying infants appear to have shut themselves off from all external stimulation including the soothing techniques of the examiner. These episodes tend to end as abruptly as they began with the exhausted infant dropping into a deep sleep.

Orientation in the Cocaine-Exposed Infant

Orientation in the NBAS refers to the infant's ability to interact actively with the outside world by attending to and responding to visual and auditory stimuli presented either singly or simultaneously. During an NBAS exam, normal drug-free newborns, with varying degrees of examiner assistance, can typically achieve repeated episodes of responsiveness to external stimuli. They can often track visual stimuli with their eyes and sometimes head and eyes. They will alert to sounds and frequently try to locate these sounds. By one month of age, most normal drug-free infants are able to respond appropriately to visual and auditory stimuli for lengthy periods of time with little or no assistance from the examiner.

The orientation abilities of newborn cocaine-exposed infants, on the other hand, are quite limited. As was mentioned earlier, many of these infants never reach an alert responsive state at all during the NBAS exam. Those infants who do reach an alert state require a great deal of examiner-induced control to do so. Some of the containment techniques commonly used both to calm and to help organize the infants are tight swaddling, use of a pacifier, hand holding, and vertical rocking. Even with this examiner assistance, most newborn cocaine-exposed infants are capable of only fleeting attention to a stimulus before they begin showing signs of distress including color changes, rapid respiration, frantic gaze aversion, and disorganized motor activity. To reduce the likelihood of an infant becoming overloaded by stimulation, the examiner should withdraw the stimulus being presented at the first signs of infant distress and allow the infant time-out to recover. If this is done, the examiner may be able to bring the infant back to respond briefly to another stimulus. For most of the newborn cocaine-exposed infants, each stimulus presented seems to have a cumulative effect towards overloading the infants so that they are less responsive to each successive stimulus. Once these infants reach their point of overstimulation, they will usually terminate the exam by either pulling down into sleep state or moving into an unavailable crying state.

By one month of age, there is a noticeable improvement in the orientation abilities of the cocaine-exposed infants, but their performance is still significantly poorer than drug-free newborns[11]. The one-month-old cocaine-exposed infants are still quite dependent upon the organizational structure provided by the examiner in the forms described above. Without this examiner assistance many of them are quickly overloaded by even mild levels of stimulation and move into an unresponsive crying state. With examiner facilitation, however, the infants are capable of responding repeatedly to stimuli for brief periods. The examiner-induced controls also seem to reduce the infants' level of excitement and disorganization enough so that they are able to utilize a variety of self-protective behaviors to gain even better control. These behaviors include such things as gaze aversion, visual locking, eye closing, and controlled motor movements. They serve not only as self-protective behaviors for the infant but as cues to the examiner to slow down the presentation of stimuli and/or allow the infant some time to reorganize. With this type of sensitive handling, many of the one-month-old cocaine-exposed infants are able to tolerate repeated responsive periods. Each additional period of responsiveness, however, seems to take such a toll on the infants' energy reserves that by the end of the exam, most of them are obviously exhausted and on the verge of losing control.

MATERNAL CHARACTERISTICS

Conversations with the cocaine-abusing mothers treated by our program and observations of their interactions with their infants have indicated that many of them are experiencing the same feelings about parenthood and demonstrating the same deficiencies in knowledge which have been seen in other programs treating drug-addicted mothers[12]. Many of the mothers experience guilt concerning the potential damage which their cocaine abuse may have done to their infant. Some of them are fearful concerning their ability to cope with and successfully meet the demands of their child. Finally, a number of the mothers appear to have unrealistic expectations about their infants' competencies stemming from a basic naivete concerning normal infant development.

When these often insecure, sometimes inadequate mothers are paired with the type of irritable, easily overloaded, unresponsive infants described earlier, it is not surprising that a number of pathological maternal – infant relationships develop. In the worst of these relationships, the mothers appear to have detached themselves almost completely from their infants. It is frequently difficult to get these mothers to comply with the developmental follow-up schedule and when they do show up for appointments, they appear very lethargic and display flat affects. During the developmental testing of their infants, the detached mothers often stare blankly at the wall or sometimes sleep. They pay little or no attention to either their infants' behavior or the feedback provided to them concerning how to better care for their infants. In a number of such cases, the mothers have withdrawn from their infants to the point that almost all of the caretaking responsibilities for the infant have had to be taken over by other family members.

Fortunately, the majority of the mothers we see do not detach themselves from their infants. Many of those who remain attached to their infants, however, experience a great deal of frustration over trying to cope with their irritable, unresponsive infants. Some of them appear to interpret their infants' attempts to shut out external stimulation as personal rejections of them as mothers. This perceived rejection may serve to confirm in some of the mothers their feelings that they are bad mothers thereby increasing any feelings of depression and worthlessness which these women might be experiencing. Other mothers seem to blame the baby for rejecting them and seem to display ambivalent and sometimes hostile feelings towards the infant.

So far we have presented a very negative view of cocaine-abusing women as mothers. It would be unfair, however, to the mothers we follow not to point out that many of them overcome considerable personal problems and become very sensitive, responsive mothers who do everything in their power to make sure that all of their infants needs are met.

IMPROVING THE MATERNAL – INFANT RELATIONSHIP

As a first step towards building a functional relationship between the cocaine-abusing mothers in our program and their infants, we have used some of the techniques which Brazelton[1] has used successfully to foster the relationship between premature infants and their parents. To date our intervention efforts have been limited to feedback given to the mothers during the administration of and directly following the NBAS exams on their infants at birth, one week, and one month of age. By using the information we gain from the NBAS, we hope to educate the mothers about the competencies and needs of their infants. We also are attempting to teach the mothers those containment and structuring techniques which will allow them to take an active role in improving the overall organization and consequently the responsiveness of their infants. By arming the mothers with specific skills to work with their infants we may increase their confidence and competence in dealing with their infants and reduce any tendency they may have to withdraw from their infants.

Our first effort to teach the mothers how to interact with their infants occurs immediately following the NBAS exam on the newborns. At this time we explain to the mother how fragile her infant is in terms of ease of overstimulation. We then describe for her the types of stimulation which seem to most easily overload her infant and the signals which the infant will emit when he/she is beginning to become over-stimulated. These signals range from early distress signals, such as yawns, sneezes, hiccoughs and grimaces, to the signs of panic, such as frantic gaze aversion, color changes, spitting up, jerky movements and crying. We explain to the mother that by reducing stimulation to the infant at the first signs of distress she can frequently avoid a crying episode. We assure the mother that when her infant engages in these distress behaviors, he/she is trying to ask for her help and not rejecting her as a mother. We also tell the mother that there will be times when nothing she does will be able to avert a crying episode in her infant. To cope with these episodes when they occur, we teach her how to use the soothing techniques of swaddling, use of pacifier, and vertical rocking to calm the infant.

Since many of the mothers in our program are concerned about possibly spoiling their infants by responding to their every cry, it is very important for the examiner to emphasize to the mother that the earlier in a crying episode she intervenes with soothing techniques, the more quickly the infant will calm down. We end the initial session by giving the mother two things to concentrate on during the first week of the baby's life: (1) keeping the infant as calm as possible using the techniques provided and, (2) taking advantage of the infant's quiet, alert states to work briefly on his responsivensss by presenting either visual or auditory stimuli, but usually not both. We explain to her that presenting a stimulus with both visual and auditory features to the infant may be more stimulating than he/she can tolerate. We also warn her to pay careful attention to the infant's cues during this orientation exercise and to use time-outs as the infant requires them.

In order to make these general instructions more concrete for the mothers, we instruct the mother to start out by trying to engage the infant face to face without speaking or moving her face around too much. If the infant is able to fix his eyes on her comfortably, then she might try talking in a quiet, rhythmic voice to the infant. At other times when the infant is focused on her, she can try moving her face slowly across the infant's visual field without speaking in order to engage the infant in visual tracking. If her infant's cues are telling the mother that human stimulation is too complex or too exciting for him/her to tolerate, we suggest that she try getting her infant to visually fix on and follow a simpler, inanimate object such as a red ball used in the NBAS. If visual stimulation of any type proves to be too much for the infant, we suggest to the mother that she can still improve her infant's tolerance for stimulation by talking in a low rhythmic voice to him/her without trying to engage him/her visually. An ideal position for this type of interaction is to have the mother hold the infant vertically against her chest, but facing away from the mother. This allows the mother to contain the infant's movements and stimulate him audially, but frees the infant from the pressure to visually engage any stimuli.

The second session with the mother occurs during the infant's one week NBAS exam. This entire exam is performed in the presence of the mother so that we can reinforce the lessons of the previous week by both describing and demonstrating them for the mother. We try to get the mother to pay particular attention to the techniques which we use to achieve alert responsiveness in her infant, the infant's distress cues, and how adjusting the presentation of stimulus materials can help keep the infant calm. We end this second session by encouraging the mother to continue to help her infant increase his/her responsiveness by presenting him/her with visual and auditory stimuli for longer and longer periods and even in combination. We warn her again, however, to use the infant's distress cues as her guide to determining how much stimulation to present to her infant in any one session. We also encourage her to use the techniques she has observed that day to help her infant avoid losing control during a session and to regain control if he has been overstimulated.

The third session with the mother occurs during the infants one month NBAS exam. Once again the mother is present for the exam and we describe for her what we are seeing in the infant, as we see it. We point out any improvements we notice in the infant's behavior and re-emphasize the necessity of using the infant's cues as a guide to when and how to stimulate the infant.

Following this assessment, we discuss with the mother the need to continue to help the infant to avoid overstimulation and complete loss of control, while at the same time gradually increasing his tolerance for stimulation and his capacity for self-control. To accomplish these goals, we once again encourage the mother to work on the infant's orientation skills during his/her calmest, wakeful periods. We encourage her to gradually increase the length of time during which she engages her infant with auditory and/or visual stimulation always using the infant's cues as the indicator of whether to continue or cease stimulation. During these times, the infant might be unwrapped (only if he/she will tolerate this) to let him get used to controlling his own body movements and to increase his tolerance for stimulation without the aid of external controls. It is important to emphasize to the mother that we are not suggesting she give up swaddling her infant altogether, but that she use it according to her infant's need for it.

SUMMARY

As mentioned earlier, our efforts at parental training have been limited to demonstrations and feedback given to the mothers during the course of and directly following our developmental evaluations of their infants. No systematic analysis of the effectiveness of the training has been completed. It is our observation, however, that the information we provide is being utilized by at least some of the mothers as judged by their descriptions of their interactions with their infants and the improvement we see in the organization and responsiveness of the infants. With many of our other mothers, however, it seems that the limited time we spend with them during the first few weeks of the infant' lives is not nearly enough both to break down their defenses and to teach them how to interact with their infant in a productive fashion. What is needed is a more comprehensive maternal training program with at least weekly sessions with a developmental specialist who could continuously fine tune and reinforce the mothers' responsiveness to their infants' cues. This should be combined with the medical, social, and emotional support which could be provided by a multi-disciplinary team of pediatricians, nurses, social workers and therapists.

REFERENCES

1. Brazelton, T.B. (1982). Behavioral assessment of the premature infant: Uses in intervention. In Klaus, M.H. and Robertson, M.O. (eds.), *Birth, Interaction and Attachment.* pp. 85–92. (Johnson and Johnson Baby Products Company)
2. Field, T.M. (1977). Effects of early separation, interactive deficits, and experimental manipulation on infant–mother face-to-face interaction. *Child Devel.*, 48, 763–71
3. Horowitz, F.D. (1984). The psychobiology of parent–offspring relations in high-risk situations. *Adv. Infancy Res.*, 3, 1–22
4. Horowitz, F.D. and Linn, P.L. (1982). The Neonatal Behavioral Assessment Scale: Assessing the behavioral repertoire of the newborn infant. *Adv. Devel. Behav. Pediatr.*, 3, 133–55
5. Lief, N.R. and Zarin-Ackerman, J. (1980). Sociocultural deprivation and its effect on the development of the child. In Bemporad, J.R. (ed.), *Child Development in Normality and Psychopathology*, pp. 362–392. (New York: Brunne/Mazel Publishers)
6. Osofsky, J.D. and Danzger, B. (1974). Relationships between neonatal characteristics and mother–infant interactions. *Devel. Psychol.*, 10(1), 124–30
7. Siegel, E. (1982). A critical examination of studies of parent–infant bonding. In Klaus, M.H. and Robertson, M.O. (eds.), *Birth, Interaction and Attachment*, pp. 51–61. (Johnson and Johnson Baby Products Company)
8. Solnit, A.J. (1984). Keynote address: Theoretical and practical aspects of risks and vulnerabilities in infancy. *Child Abuse Neglect*, 8, 133–44
9. Brazelton, T.B. (1984). *Neonatal Behavioral Assessment Scale.* (Philadelphia: J.B. Lippincott Co.)
10. Chasnoff, I.J., Burns, W.J., Schnoll, S.H. and Burns, K.A. (1985). Cocaine use in pregnancy. *N. Engl. J. Med.*, 313, 666–9
11. Griffith, D., Chasnoff, I., Dirkes, K. and Burns, K. (1988). Neurobehavioral development of cocaine-exposed infants in the first month of life. *Pediatr. Res.* (Abstract in press)
12. Lief, N.R. (1985). The drug user as a parent. *Int. J. Addict.*, 20(1), 63–97

9

Motor Assessment and Parent Education Beyond the Newborn Period

Jane W Schneider

Most of the information about the effects of *in utero* drug exposure on developmental progress has been confined primarily to the newborn period[1-4]. Specifically, the area of motor development has not been adequately described for the period of early infancy. Previously infants born to drug-using mothers were tested using the Motor Scale of the Bayley Scales of Infant Development (BSID). Results showed that the motor behavior of drug-exposed infants fell within the normal range through two years of age[5]. These findings were surprising to the staff working with the drug-exposed infants since their intuitive clinical judgement was that these infants did not compare to normal non-drug-exposed infants of the same age. They felt that a difference in development did indeed exist, even though the BSID was not able to detect one. A closer look at the Motor Scale of the BSID[6] finds it to have few items for each age range. Also it provides more of a check list of motor development rather than a qualitative assessment.

To attempt to document the motor behavior of drug-exposed infants we began to utilize a test called the Movement Assessment of Infants (MAI)[7]. The MAI is designed to evaluate the categories of muscle tone, primitive reflexes, automatic reactions and volitional movement in the first year of life.

The **muscle tone** section of the test evaluates the ability of the infant's muscles to counteract gravity in a variety of positions. **Reflex testing** is similar to standard neurological testing although scoring of these items is much more qualitative. For example, besides determining the presence or absence of a primitive reflex, the MAI assesses how much the reflex dominates the infant's movement patterns. The **automatic reactions** category evaluates the development of righting and equilibrium reactions. Responses to auditory and visual stimulation, and gross and fine motor development are assessed in the **volitional movement** section of the test.

The MAI provides, at 4 months of age, an assessment of risk for motor dysfunction using an *a priori* profile of normal 4-month-old motor behavior. Although the MAI is not normed, reliability and validity studies have been reported for the current *a priori* profile. Inter-rater reliability has been reported as 0.72 and 0.90 or above[7,8]. Predictive validity with a sample of 246 high-risk infants found significant correlations of MAI total-risk scores with developmental evaluations at one and two years of age[9]. A recent study found that the MAI was more than twice as sensitive as the Bayley Motor Scale in detecting early signs of cerebral palsy[10]. We felt that the Movement Assessment of Infants would be a useful motor assessment tool with cocaine-exposed infants as well.

We began testing infants exposed to cocaine using the MAI in 1985 and have compared these infants to 50 non-drug exposed infants selected by a sample of convenience from the Chicago area. Demographics of the two groups are shown in Table 9.1. Sex and race were the only demographics variables examined because previous studies have shown no significant development differences in the first year of life based on sociocultural status or maternal educational level[11,12]. Both groups however, contained infants from low-income families.

Table 9.1 Demographic data

	Sex				Race					
	Male		Female		Black		White		Other	
	n	%	n	%	n	%	n	%	n	%
Cocaine-exposed infants	15	50	15	50	20	66	8	27	2	7
Non-drug-exposed infants	25	50	25	50	20	40	24	48	6	12

An infant's exposure to cocaine was determined either by the mother's report or urine toxicology screen. Lack of *in utero* drug exposure was determined from the infants medical record. Infants in both groups were tested on the MAI at 4 months corrected age ± one week. All of the infants were full term with the exception of four infants in the cocaine-exposed group whose gestation ranged from 33 to 37 weeks. Both groups of infants had had no serious medical problems or major congenital anomalies and were healthy at the time of testing. Parental consent was obtained for all subjects. The MAI was administered to the infants in the presence of their parent(s). The test required 30–45 minutes to complete. Each child was evaluated through observation or direct handling on the 65 MAI items.

The MAI was administered by one examiner and scoring of the MAI was completed as described in the test manual[7]. Each possible score for every item on the MAI has been designated normal or questionable for a normal four-month-old infant. For each questionable score, one high-risk point is given. High-risk score points are added from each test section to determine the total risk score. Based on previous data, the authors of the MAI have designated total risk scores of 0–7 as 'no risk', 8–13 'questionable risk', and greater than 13 as 'high risk'[7].

The MAI test form utilized did not contain the *a priori* profile. Only after the tests were administered and scored, were scores checked against the profile. This delay in determining total risk scores was adopted to minimize examiner bias during testing. The examiner was not blind to the babies' involvement in our chemical dependence program, but did not know the type of drug abused by the mother. Only cocaine-exposed infants were included in this study. Consequently, eighteen additional infants were tested who did not meet the criteria for the study, based on corrected age at time of testing or type of drug used by the mother.

Before discussing the results of our study, I'd like to describe some key characteristics of normal four-month-old motor behavior. First, in supine, four-month-olds are very active. They can reach out easily and grasp objects offered to them. They bring their hands easily to midline and finger one hand with the other. The infants lower extremities are also very active. They can flex and extend their legs and kick reciprocally. The infants flex their legs in order to begin playing with and exploring their knees and feet. This is an important part of learning and contributes to the proper development of body image. While some four-month-olds have developed enough trunk rotation to roll from their back to their stomachs, most have developed enough flexibility to at least roll to their sides. Flexibility is a key descriptor of four-month-old motor development. They are developing control of both the flexor and extensor muscle groups without being dominated by either one. Even though a four-month-old cannot stand independently, when held in supported standing, this flexibility is seen by a relaxed standing posture that incorporates both flexor and extensor muscle control.

The attempt of our study was to see how the motor patterns of cocaine-exposed infants compared to non-drug-exposed infants. First the total risk score derived from the MAI was not comparable, with the cocaine-exposed infants scoring significantly worse (Figure 9.1). Also, the cocaine-exposed infants scored significantly more poorly on the muscle tone, primitive reflexes and volitional movement categories (Figures 9.2, 9.3 and 9.4). Only the automatic reaction section of the test showed no significant difference between the groups.

Looking at the items individually, the groups scored differently on 19 of the 65 MAI items. Table 9.2 lists the test sections and items where significant differences were found. For all the items listed, with the exception of A14, 'placing of hands', cocaine-exposed infants scored lower than the non-drug exposed infants. Finally placement of infants within previously established ranges of risk scores revealed a significant difference between the groups (Figure 9.5). While 72% of the non-drug-exposed 4-month-olds fell into the no-risk category, only 27% of the cocaine-exposed infants are designated 'no risk'. Conversely, only 2% (1 out of 50) of the control infants fell into the 'high risk' range, while 43% (13 out of 30) of the cocaine-exposed infants would be considered at high risk for motor developmental dysfunction. Our findings suggest that the relative risk for motor developmental delay in cocaine-exposed infants is approximately 40 times higher than for infants not exposed to drugs *in utero*.

While *in utero* cocaine exposure does not affect the motor development of all exposed infants, it appears to have a profound effect on others. Cocaine-exposed infants have been noted clinically to display increased extensor muscle tone[13]. This finding was also supported in our study by the high-risk scores in the significant differences on 6 of the 10 muscle tone items (see Table 9.2). In contrast to the normal 4-month-olds, the cocaine-exposed

Table 9.2 Item by item comparison

Category	Item no.	Item name
Muscle tone	T 1	Consistency
	T 2	Extensibility
	T 4	Posture in supine
	T 6	Posture in prone suspended
	T 8	Distribution variation
	T 9	Summary of tone in extremities
Primitive reflexes	R 1	Tonic labyrinthine reflex-supine
	R 6	Tremulousness
	R 10	Neonatal positive support
	R 11	Walking reflex
	R 14	Summary of primitive reflexes
Automatic reactions	A 5	Rotation in trunk
	A 6	Equilibrium reactions in prone
	A 8	Equilibrium reactions vertical suspension
	A 14	Placing of hands
Volitional movement	V 4	Vocalization
	V 17	Active use of hips
	V 25	Summary of volitional movements

$p < 0.01$

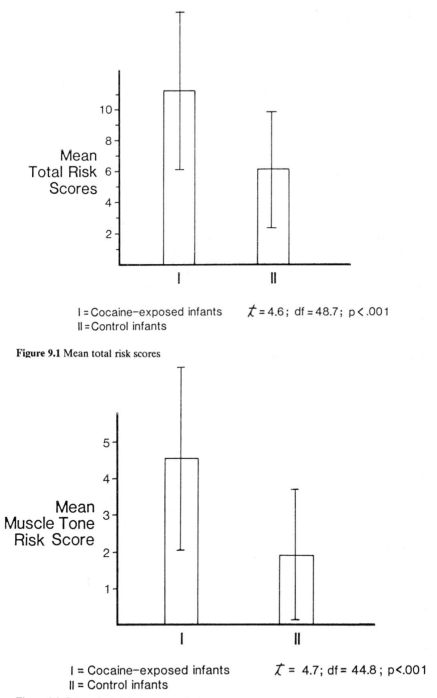

I = Cocaine-exposed infants t = 4.6; df = 48.7; p < .001
II = Control infants

Figure 9.1 Mean total risk scores

I = Cocaine-exposed infants t = 4.7; df = 44.8; p<.001
II = Control infants

Figure 9.2 Categorical risk score: muscle tone

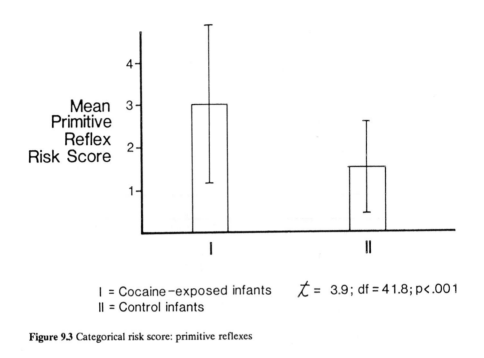

I = Cocaine-exposed infants $t = 3.9$; df = 41.8; p<.001
II = Control infants

Figure 9.3 Categorical risk score: primitive reflexes

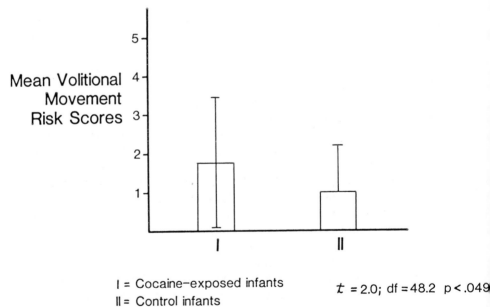

I = Cocaine-exposed infants $t = 2.0$; df = 48.2 p<.049
II = Control infants

Figure 9.4 Categorical risk score: volitional movements

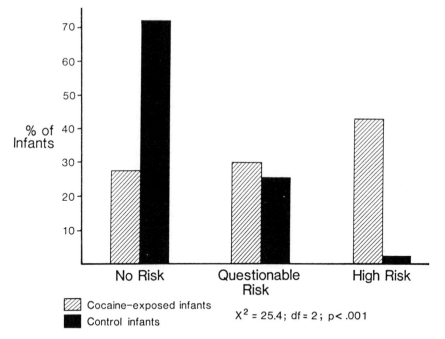

Figure 9.5 Placement of infants within risk categories

infants often lie supine in excessively extended postures and have difficulty moving their limbs against gravity. Their movements are often jerky and stiff, and the variability in their movement patterns is diminished.

The results of our study suggest that cocaine-exposed infants show delayed integration of some of the primitive reflexes. Tremors, especially of their upper extremities, were frequently noted during the evaluation. They demonstrated an exaggerated positive support reaction that was characterized by stiff extension of the trunk and legs and weight bearing on their toes. The primitive walking reflex, usually integrated at two months of age, could still be elicited easily at four months of age.

Cocaine-exposed infants showed differences in volitional movements when compared to normal infants. They were less able to round their buttocks off the supporting surface or kick reciprocally. The normal visual and manual exploration of their lower limbs was often not possible for the cocaine-exposed infants due to the increased extensor muscle tone which limited their lower extremity flexibility.

In general, cocaine-exposed infants have more difficulty moving against the forces of gravity and display more immature movement patterns than non-drug-exposed infants. While this is certainly an important outcome of our developmental assessment, equally important is the parent education that occurs during the evaluation session.

The purpose of our parent education is two-fold; to enhance normal infant development and to foster a strong parent–infant relationship.

Parent education occurs through both direct and indirect means. We believe that much indirect education can occur by having the parent(s) observe and participate in the evaluation session. Parents are able to observe the examiner interacting with their infant, and modeling appropriate contingent behavior. That is, the parent observes the examiner pausing to allow the child time to respond to each request, and assisting the child only when necessary to complete a task. In addition, as the therapist handles the child during the evaluation, the parent observes appropriate ways to deal with their child physically. For example, many cocaine-exposed infants with increased muscled tone must be moved slowly to avoid further increasing their tone.

Finally the evaluation is an opportune time to highlight strengths and weaknesses that their child possesses. When a child calms easily, for example, the examiner can comment on this to the parent. Often an infant is able to accomplish something that is unexpected to the parent. In the four-month-old infants, this is often sitting momentarily without support. Observing their child accomplish a new, yet unknown, skill is very reinforcing to the parent and the parent–child relationship. On the other hand, weaknesses, such as increased tremors in the arms and hands, are also pointed out to parents. It is explained how these abnormal signs might interfere with normal activities, (In this case, tremors may interfere with reaching.) By offering signs of their child's strengths as well as weaknesses, the examiner is seen by the parents as presenting a more realistic view of their child.

Evaluating the infant's motor abilities also provides many opportunities for direct parent education. In supine, cocaine-exposed infants show increased extensor tone. This tone causes decreased pelvic mobility and limits the infant from lifting the legs up to play with his knees or to kick reciprocally. Parents can be taught to lift the infant's pelvis up and flex the legs toward the chest, enabling the infant to overcome the extensor tone and to begin increased kicking movements with the lower extremities. From this position of supine flexion, the lower extremities can be rotated from side to side to further decrease extensor tone (Figure 9.3). Parents should be warned against leaving their infants in supine for long periods, since increased extensor tone and the effects of gravity make movement difficulty in this position.

Other forms of relaxation can be taught to parents, expecially for those infants who become irritable when handled, a common finding in cocaine-exposed infants.

Initially an infant may need to be swaddled in a blanket in a semiflexed position. The warmth from the blanket appears to caues inhibition of motor behavior[14]. In addition, the flexed position breaks up the extensor tone, decreases tremors and overshooting, and facilitates normal hand-to-mouth activity. In conjunction with swaddling, slow rocking may be necessary to calm the infant. Studies have shown that such vestibular proprioceptive stimulation frequently has the immediate effect of arresting crying, reducing irritability, and bringing the infant to a visually alert state[15]. This produces a sense of effectiveness in the caregiver and allows both infant and caregiver to be prepared for social interaction. While vestibular-proprioceptive input appears to have a strong effect on the infant's motor control, other forms of slow rhythmical input (e.g. visual, auditory, tactile) could be used to 'pacify' the infant[15]. Once the infant has become calm, he or she can be held in the *en face* (face-to-face) position to encourage visual following vocalization, and playful interaction with the caregiver.

Repeated demonstrations of positioning and handling techniques to relax and begin interacting with the infant, as well as return demonstration, by the parents, are all part of the educational process.

Another unique way of handling the cocaine-exposed infant to reduce irritability and improve motor control is the use of neonatal hydrotherapy. Sweeney[17,18] has utilized hydrotherapy in an intensive care nursery setting and has found it to be effective in improving posture, muscle tone, behavioral state, and feeding behaviors in premature infants. These outcomes are also appropriate for cocaine-exposed infants.

While swaddling, rocking, and other methods of calming may initially be necessary, it is important to teach parents to use these methods only as needed and to begin to withdraw these additional techniques as soon as possible so that the infant learns to gain control over his or her own state. For example, swaddling may initially be necessary frequently when the infant is handled. As the infant responds more to calming measures and begins to show self-calming abilities, swaddling should only be utilized when the infant seems unable to respond without this intervention.

Parents are frequently interested in play positions for their infants. Unfortunately they often turn too quickly to devices such as baby walkers or jumpers. Use of assistive devices such as jumpers and walkers should be discouraged. Parents should be informed that thousands of injuries each year are related to the use of these devices*. As importantly, infants placed in these devices are not 'exercising' their muscles appropriately, since they do

---

* Interestingly, the Canadian Medical Association has recently requested that their government ban the sale of walkers altogether because of frequent injuries to children[19].

not yet have the ability to hold themselves in proper postural alignment when placed in the upright position. The leg actions of a baby in a walker have little relationship to walking skills[20]. Rather than training an infant to walk, the walker may actually impede progress by inhibiting the infant from crawling around[21]. Walkers encourage the hypertonic infants (like the cocaine-exposed infants) to further increase their extensor tone by pushing their feet against the floor and arching their trunks backwards[22].

Prone is a good position for infants to develop antigravity extensor strength. Because cocaine-exposed infants have a preponderance of extensor tone, they usually enjoy this position and perform well in it. The infants should be encouraged to move in prone by placing colorful stimulating toys beside them, promting pivoting in the trunk to reach the toys.

Rather than lengthy exercise programs and complicated instructions to follow, parents need practical advise on how to best encourage their child's normal motor development. Parents can be taught to carry their infants in a way that will control the infants muscle tone while facilitating head and trunk control as well as the ability to reach and grasp objects. Rather than specific 'do's and don'ts' parents can be taught to assess their infant's response to handling as a guideline. For example, some cocaine-exposed infants may be more sensitive to quick rough movement (rough-house play) and may respond by stiffening their bodies or crying. This response should indicate that this type of play is too stimulating for their infant to handle and should be replaced by slow gentle swinging through the air.

Most importantly, parent education will change as the needs of their infant's change.

While many cocaine-exposed infants may not require intensive physical therapy, monthly sessions may be necessary to demonstrate developmentally appropriate activities and to teach parents new handling skills. As always, return demonstrations from parents are important to confirm their level of skill and understanding.

In summary, the effects of *in utero* cocaine exposure on motor development in infancy are only now being explored. Qualitative motor assessment of the at-risk infant provides valuable information about the effects of this exposure. The strength of any perinatal chemical dependence program lies in combining research fact-finding activities with clinical intervention. During physical therapy motor assessment, in addition to data collection, intervention is possible through both direct and indirect parent education concerning their infants developmental progress.

REFERENCES

1. Chasnoff, I.J., Burns, K.A. and Burns, W.J. (1987). Cocaine use in pregnancy: perinatal morbidity and mortality. *Neurotoxicol. Teratol.*, **9**, 291–3
2. MacGregor, S.N., Keith, L.G., Chasnoff, I.J., Rosner, M.A., Chisum, G.M., Shaw, P. and Minegue, J.P. (1987). Cocaine use in pregnancy: adverse perinatal outcome. *Am. J. Obstet. Gynecol.*, **157**, 686–90
3. Oro, A.S. and Dixon, S.D. (1987). Perinatal cocaine and methamphetamine exposure: maternal and neonatal correlates. *J. Pediatr.*, **111**, 571–8
4. Ryan, L., Ehrlich, S. and Finnegan, L. (1987). Cocaine abuse in pregnancy: effects on the fetus and newborn. *Neurotoxicol. Teratol.*, **9**, 295–9
5. Chasnoff, I.J., Burns, K.A., Burns, W.J. and Schnoll, S.H. (1986). Prenatal drug exposure: effects on neonatal and infant growth and development. *Neurobehav. Toxicol. Teratol.*, **8**, 357–62
6. Bayley, N. (1969). *Manual for the Bayley Scales of Infant Development.* (New York: The Physiological Corporation)
7. Chandler, L.S., Andrews, M.S. and Swanson, M.W. (1980). *Movement assessment of infants, a Manual.* (Rolling Bay, WA: Movement Assessment of Infants)
8. Harris, S.R., Haley, S., Tada, W.L. and Swanson, M.W. (1984). Reliability of observational measures of the Movement Assessment of Infants. *Phys. Ther.*, **64**, 471–5
9. Harris, S.R., Swanson, S.W., Chandler, T.S., Andrews, M.S., Sells, C.J., Robinson, N.M. and Bennett, F.C. (1984). Predictive validity of the Movement Assessment of Infants. *Devel. Behav. Pediatr.*, **5**, 336–42
10. Harris, S.R. (1987). Early detection of cerebral palsy: sensitivity and specificity of two motor assessment tools. *J. Perinatol.*, **7**, 11–15
11. Ireton, H., Thwing, E. and Gravem, H. (1970). Infant mental development and neurological status, family socioeconomic status and intelligence at age four. *Child Devel.*, **41**, 937–45
12. Knoblock, H. and Pasamanick, B. (1960). An evaluation of the consistency and predictive value of the 40 week Gesell Developmental Schedule. In Shagass, C. and Pasamanick, B. (eds.) *Child Development and Child Psychiatry, Psychiatric Research Reports*, **13**, 10–31. (Washington, DC: American Psychiatric Association)
13. Schneider, J.W. and Chasnoff, I.J. (1987). Cocaine abuse during pregnancy: its effects on infant motor development – a clinical perspective. *Topics Acute Care Trauma Rehab.*, **2**, 599–69
14. Umphred, D.A. and McCromack, G.L. (1985). Classification of common facilitory and inhibitory treatment techniques. In Umphred, D.A. (ed.) *Neurological Rehabilitation.* (St Louis: Mosby)
15. Korner, A. (1984). Interconnections between sensory and affective development in early infancy. In *Zero to Three*, **5**, 1–6. (Washington DC: Bulletin of the National Center for Clinical Infant Programs)
16. Wilhelm, I.J. (1984). The neurologically suspect neonate. In Cambell, S.K. (ed.) *Pediatric Neurologic Physical Therapy.* (New York: Churchill Livingstone)
17. Sweeney, J.K. (1985). Neonates at developmental risk. In Umphred, D.A. (ed.) *Neurological Rehabilitation.* (St. Louis: Mosby)
18. Sweeney, J.K. (1983). Neonatal hydrotherapy: An adjunct to developmental intervention in an intensive care nursery setting. *Phys. Occup. Ther. Pediatr.*, **3**, 20
19. Newsbriefs (1987). Ban sale of baby walkers, CMA urges. *Can. Med. Assoc. J.*, **136**, 57
20. Editors of Consumer Guide (1979). *The Complete Baby Book.* (New York: Simon & Schuster)
21. Various (1987). Notes from readers: more on infant walkers. *Pediatric Notes*, **26**, 46
22. Simpkiss, M.J. and Raikes, A.S. (1972). Problems resulting from the excessive use of baby-walkers and baby bouncers. *Lancet*, **1**, 747

10

FAS: Clinical Perspectives and Prevention

Lyn Weiner and Barbara A Morse

INTRODUCTION

Concern about the effects of parental consumption of alcohol at the time of conception and during gestation can be traced back to ancient civilizations[1]. Burton[2] cited Aristotle's *Problemata*, "foolish, drunken, or hare-brain women for the most part bring forth children like themselves, morose and languid". Interest in alcohol's effects on pregnancy waxed and waned over the years, influenced as much by sociological and moralistic factors as by scientific findings.

Epidemiologic and experimental research accumulated in the early 1900s, documenting the relationship between parental drinking and adverse pregnancy outcome. In 1920, when the 18th amendment was ratified and Prohibition went into effect, research on alcohol virtually disappeared. Following the repeal of prohibition in 1933, scientists discounted the early studies because of their primitive experimental techniques and moralistic overtones.

The notion that heavy maternal drinking is detrimental to offspring regained scientific status when Lemoine *et al.*[3] and Jones and Smith[4] observed a common pattern of malformations in offspring of chronic alcoholic women. Jones and Smith coined the term 'fetal alcohol syndrome' (FAS) to define a pattern of prenatal and postnatal growth deficiency, developmental delay or mental retardation, microcephaly, fine motor dysfunction and a characteristic facial dysmorphology. The initial publications describing FAS stimulated case reports from around the world, which have been followed by thousands of clinical, epidemiologic and experimental studies[5]. The body of findings has shown that ethanol and its metabolites have the potential to alter the growth and development of the embryo and fetus. Clinical observations have been confirmed by experimental studies which show structural, growth and behavioral defects in association with maternal ethanol exposure. Alcohol consumption is now widely acknow-

127

ledged to be a risk factor for adverse pregnancy outcome. Understanding the mechanisms which underlie alcohol's actions allows the development of effective prevention techniques. Clinical intervention with problem drinking women represents a powerful strategy for the prevention of alcohol-related birth defects.

DIAGNOSIS OF FAS

In 1980 the Fetal Alcohol Study Group of the Research Society on Alcoholism agreed on the importance of standard minimal criteria for the diagnosis of FAS[6]. They recommended that the diagnosis be made when there are signs in each of three categories:

1. prenatal and/or postnatal growth retardation (weight, length, and/or head circumference below the tenth percentile);

2. central nervous system involvement (signs of neurologic abnormality, developmental delay, or intellectual impairment);

3. characteristic facial dysmorphology with at least two of the following signs:
   a) microcephaly,
   b) micro-opthalmia and/or short palpebral fissures,
   c) poorly developed philtrum, thin upper lip, or flattening of the maxillary area.

In addition to the diagnostic signs, children with FAS have a higher frequency of non-specific malformations than the general population.

FAS is a clinically recognizable syndrome; however, the diagnosis cannot be made on the basis of any single distinctive feature or biochemical, chromosomal, or pathological test. All alcohol-related birth defects are non-specific and can be caused by factors other than alcohol. Since there are a limited number of responses to stress, abnormalities which result from exposure to one or more teratogens can be similar. The specific nature of abnormalities is associated with the developmental stage at the time of exposure as well as to the properties of the teratogen. A careful history is needed to differentiate alcohol-related birth defects from those due to other teratogens. The combination of growth retardation, central nervous system involvement and facial dysmorphology is not unique to FAS. It is similar to signs seen in other disorders, including fetal hydantoin syndrome which occurs in children of epileptic women who have taken anticonvulsant drugs[7].

In some cases the diagnosis of FAS can be made in the neonate. In others, one or two years will pass before postnatal growth retardation and developmental or intellectual delays are recognized. The characteristic facial dysmorphology is more easily discerned after the newborn period. In severe cases, dysmorphic features in the newborn are sufficiently distinct to be identified, but diagnosis is impeded when cases are mild. In a study at Boston City Hospital, four out of five children with FAS were not identified at birth but were subsequently recognized during routine follow-up care[8].

FAS has been reported in scientific literature worldwide and occurs in all ethnic groups and at all socio-economic levels. All reported cases have been born to chronic alcoholic women who drank heavily during pregnancy. Not all children of women drinking abusively demonstrate FAS. Case reports suggest incidence rates among alcohol-dependent women between 33%[9] and 40%[10]. Prospective studies suggest markedly lower rates, between 2.5%[11] and 10%[8]. A higher frequency (1 in 25) has been reported among American Indians living on reservations[12]. Incidence figures for the total population are reported to be 1.9 per thousand live births[13].

Alcohol's effects on fetal development encompass a wide range with the FAS at the far end of the spectrum. Some children exposed to alcohol *in utero* exhibit components of the syndrome in the absence of the full FAS. When one or two signs occur, the terms 'possible fetal alcohol effects' (FAE), or 'alcohol-related birth defects' are used. The incidence rate of FAE is difficult to determine as the symptoms are not specific. However, it is likely that FAE occurs three times more frequently than FAS.

Growth Disturbances

The most common sign of alcohol's effects on fetal development is retarded growth in weight, length and head circumference, both *in utero* and during childhood. Although growth retardation is associated with a number of maternal risk factors, the triad of FAS identifies a subgroup of infants with characteristics rarely found in association with other risk factors. The observed growth retardation is not a reflection of prematurity; infants with FAS are significantly smaller than non-affected infants after adjustment for gestational age. Growth retardation persists even when nutrition is adequate and the environment is stable[3,14]. Catch-up growth has been observed only among children with milder forms of FAS.

In some clinical programs, length has been observed to be more profoundly affected than weight[15], while others have observed that length and weight are equally diminished[3]. Growth deficiencies observed in adolescents demonstrate unique weight-for-height ages[16]. The short, skinny stature of early childhood changes to short, stocky stature following puberty.

2 Facial Dysmorphology

The distinctive facial dysmorphology of children with FAS most often involves the eyes, nose, lip and mid-face, but can also affect the forehead, chin and ears. The eyes are small, with short palpebral fissures (eye openings), epicanthal folds, ptosis (drooping eye lids) and strabismus (crossed eyes). The nose is often short and upturned with a low nasal bridge. The maxillary area is flat. The upper lip is thin, the Cupid's Bow is absent. The philtrum, two ridges between the nasal septum and upper lip, is poorly developed. The area between the nose and upper lips appears elongated. In some cases, the forehead seems to bulge and the mandible is under-developed. Occasionally the ears are low-set with posterior rotation[17-20].

Dysmorphologists demonstrated the importance of carefully observing subtle differences in the mid-face and eyes. Most of these characteristics represent growth failure in the mid-face which may reflect abnormal brain growth[17]. Microcephaly, a failure of skull growth, also indicates small brain size.

3 Central Nervous System Anomalies

Disturbances to the central nervous system (CNS) are the most serious consequencs of exposure to high concentrations of alcohol *in utero*. The effects manifest themselves in several ways. Delays in mental and motor development, hyperactivity, altered sleep patterns, feeding problems, language dysfunction, and perceptual problems have all been reported consistently among children whose mothers were drinking heavily during pregnancy[5,21]. Some of these symptoms have been observed in the absence of facial dysmorphology or growth retardation.

Longitudinal studies of children with FAS from around the world report a mean IQ score between 70 and 89 using age-specific tests[22-24]. Individual scores cover a broader range, from a low of 16 to a high of 130. Retardation is greatest and chance for improvement least in those children with the most severe dysmorphology and the lowest birthweights.

Examinations of less severely dysmorphic children demonstrate improvement over time. Spohr and Steinhausen[23] have reported a follow-up study of children with FAS, conducting initial examinations on 71 (mean age 4.4) and re-examination three to four years later on 56. They observed a striking reduction in the severity of morphological damage and the total number of malformations over time. Neurological examinations of 19 children utilizing EEG recordings showed a distinct improvement. Fewer children were receiving both in- and outpatient care for a number of symptoms, including eating problems, clumsiness, impaired concentration, mood and phobias. Although no increase in the frequency of symptoms occurred, some symptoms persisted, especially hyperactivity. Children who had initial IQ scores of less than 70 or greater than 115 showed no change three to four years later, but some with middle range scores improved significantly. Educational status also improved.

Other researchers have observed that learning abilities improved in children with a reduction in neurologic symptoms, such as hyperactivity and hyperexcitability[25-27]. In some cases the improvement was attributed to a specific intervention; in others improvement was tied to the passage of time. Aronson and Olegard[28] have reported that parents of alcohol-exposed children perceive their children to be more normal at ages three to four than they had been earlier. Test results confirmed a catch-up at these ages, although at ages five and six the disabilities were more pronounced once again.

Hyperactivity has been consistently reported as the most persistent behavioral disturbance[16,23] and can present a serious obstacle to learning and school performance. When combined with attention deficits, perceptual problems and language delays, the determination of learning ability is also compromised. Early identification and intervention for specific delays have the best chance of maximizing development for children with alcohol-related birth defects. Intervention programs in Germany and Sweden have reported progress using individual instruction in a consistent supportive environment[25,28]. Parent training which focuses on teaching techniques to stimulate children and help them adapt to their functional disabilities is also an effective therapeutic strategy.

The damage to the CNS may be further complicated by a home in which one or both parents is alcoholic. Dynamic interactions within the infant–caretaker system can be altered by the continuing effects of alcohol on both mother and child. Child rearing is more successful in a stable and consistent environment, often lacking in alcoholic homes. Complex interactions of environmental stress, inadequate parenting, lack of enrichment, and other associated risk factors can all contribute to poor development. Yet, case reports suggest that the prognosis for children with FAS need not be so pessimistic. Recognition of the constitutional bases of behavior and learning problems can facilitate the adoption of appropriate treatment for the child. Recognition of alcohol problems in parents and their effects on child development can facilitate treatment for families and contribute to a more optimistic prognosis for everyone.

Associated Non-Specific Morphologic Abnormalities

Like other teratogenic agents, alcohol is associated with a spectrum of malformations. Case reports of FAS patients have noted abnormalities involving almost every organ system, including the heart, face, genitalia, liver, skeleton, muscles, kidney, skin, brain and immune system[5]. These abnormalities may occur in isolation or in combination. A partial list of the anomalies which have been reported is displayed in Table 10.1.

Table 10.1 Morphologic abnormalities

Eyes	Epicanthal folds, strabismus, ptosis, hypoplastic retinal vessels
Mouth	Poor suck, cleft lip, cleft palate, small teeth
Ears	Deafness
Skeleton	Radioulnar synostosis, fusion of cervical vertebrae, retarded bone growth
Heart	Atrial and ventricular septal defects, Tetralogy of Fallot, patent ductus arteriosis
Kidney	Renal hypoplasia, hydronephrosis, urogenital sinus
Liver	Extrahepatic biliary atresia, hepatic fibrosis
Immune system	Increased infections – otitis media, upper respiratory infections, immune deficiencies
Tumors	Non-specific neoplasms
Skin	Abnormal palmar creases, irregular hair, whorls

Some epidemiological studies have reported a small but statistically significant increase in the incidence of morphologic abnormalities among children of heavy drinkers[8,18-20]. However, neither case reports nor epidemiologic studies demonstrate a unique and consistent pattern of associated abnormalities other than the diagnostic signs of FAS. The multiplicity of effects suggests that alcohol can alter development at every gestational stage. In all cases, the magnitude of the abnormalities correlates with the severity of the primary diagnostic criteria of FAS.

ALCOHOL'S ACTIONS

Clinical and experimental research findings point to multiple mechanisms which underlie alcohol's effects on fetal growth and development[5]. Alcohol in high concentrations modifies cell functions throughout the body, affecting all organ systems. Direct and indirect actions have been observed on the maternal – placental – fetal system. Biochemical and pathophysiologic effects of ethanol and its metabolite, acetaldehyde, can alter fetal development by disrupting cell differentiation and growth. Alcohol-induced alterations in maternal physiology and in the intermediate metabolism of carbohydrates, proteins and fats can alter the environment in which the fetus develops. Chronic exposure to high doses of alcohol can interfere with the passage of amino acid across the placenta and with the incorporation of amino acids into proteins[29]. The complete FAS results from the cumulative actions of high blood alcohol concentrations on the maternal – placental – fetal system throughout pregnancy.

Variability occurs in the nature and extent of the abnormalities seen in children exposed to alcohol *in utero*. It has been estimated that 2 – 10% of pregnancies complicated by alcohol produce children with FAS; another 30 – 40% have some adverse effects[13]. The differences are related to several factors, including dose levels, chronicity of alcohol use, gestational stage and duration of exposure, and sensitivity of fetal tissue.

MEDIATING FACTORS

Dose

The dose of alcohol to which the fetus is exposed is directly related to maternal blood alcohol concentration. Alcohol reaches the fetus through the process of diffusion, crossing the placental membranes easily in both directions at a rate dependent on the concentration gradient. Following ingestion, the maternal BAC rises rapidly while the fetal BAC lags behind[30]. Alcohol diffuses from the maternal system to the fetal system until they reach equilibrium; then the alcohol diffuses from the fetal circulation back into the maternal circulation. Since alcohol dehydrogenase in the fetal liver is immature and has limited capacity, the fetus is dependent on the maternal system to metabolize the alcohol. As the mother's liver metabolizes the alcohol, both the maternal and fetal BACs drop. Maximum concentrations occur later in the fetus than in the mother and do not reach as high a peak. Although the fetal BAC peaks at a lower point than that of the mother, the fetal BAC is slightly higher than the maternal BAC as they both approach zero. When the mother drinks continuously and maintains a relatively steady BAC, the difference between the maternal and fetal BAC is small.

Dose response has been explored in a few studies to test whether the magnitude of the effect increases with dose and if there is a threshold of effect. Early experimental studies with the beagle dog model demonstrated a clear dose – response effect[31]. Growth retardation and stillbirths occurred with exposure to the equivalent of 9 drinks twice a day (maternal BAC = 173 mg/dl); higher doses (maternal BAC = 205 mg/dl) were associated with stillbirths and resorptions. No effects were seen with lower doses (maternal

BAC = 101 mg/dl). Decreased birthweights and increased anomalies have also been reported in a dose-related manner in the rodent[32,33].

There are indications of a threshold for alcohol's effect as is commonly seen with other teratogens. Intraperitoneal administration of high doses of alcohol was related to weight reduction in rats while low doses were not[34]. Embryotoxic effects of alcohol were observed in rats *in vitro* only when alcohol concentrations reached those found in intoxicated humans, and they increased in direct relation to alcohol concentrations[35]. Rat pups exposed to $1-2$ g kg^{-1} day^{-1} showed minimal effects on growth which were attributed to decreased food intake[36]. Doses of 4 g kg^{-1} day^{-1} (maternal BAC of $150-200$ mg percent) was associated with growth retardation and behavioral problems, but there was catch-up growth by day 21 postpartum[37]. Permanent growth retardation and behavioral anomalies occurred with exposure to 6 g kg^{-1} day^{-1} (maternal BAC of $200-270$ mg percent). In newborn rat pups doses between 6 and 6.5 g kg^{-1} day^{-1} produced microcephaly[38]. Doses below 6 g kg^{-1} did not reduce brain size. Death occurred with doses over 7 g kg^{-1}. Peak BAC rather than alcohol dose has been demonstrated to be the critical factor in reducing brain growth in the rat[39].

Clinically, the impact of a range of drinking patterns on fetal growth has been investigated in prospective and retrospective studies conducted worldwide in the past 15 years. The relationship between heavy drinking and/or alcohol abuse and intrauterine growth retardation has been observed repeatedly[8,40-43]. Some research groups report lower birthweights in association with moderate levels of drinking as well[44,45]. Others show no association between alcohol consumption and fetal outcome[46-49].

A dose-response relationship has also been demonstrated between alcohol exposure and other adverse outcomes[50]. The severity and frequency of anatomic abnormalities (craniofacial, morphologic, and skeletal) increased with dose. Risk was greatest with consumption of more than 3 ounces of absolute alcohol a day (6 standard drinks). At lower levels, the association was less clear. A review of clinical findings in the Sixth Special Report to Congress[51] concludes that heavy drinking is detrimental and that the effects from low doses may be real, but are so small that they are difficult to measure.

Outcome is associated not only with the amount of alcohol consumed, but also with the chronicity of maternal alcoholism. High morbidity and mortality rates have been reported among mothers of FAS children. In a review of 245 cases, 75% of the mothers were dead or missing from alcohol-related problems within five years of the birth of their babies[52]. Majewski[22] observed that the severity of FAS depended on the state of maternal alcoholism and not on the absolute amount of alcohol consumed. The more severely affected children were born to women in the crucial or chronic stages of alcoholism (as defined by Jellinek[53]). Affected children who were born to women in the early stage of alcoholism were all diagnosed as having mild cases of FAS. Abel and Sokol[13] have reported that a positive MAST score (which reflects alcohol addiction) is more strongly associated with adverse outcome than dose.

Gestational Stage

Vulnerability of particular organ systems may be greatest at the time of their most rapid cell division. During the first trimester, effects of high concentrations of alcohol on cell membrane and cell migration can disturb embryonic organization of tissue, resulting in morphologic abnormalities. Throughout pregnancy, disturbances in the metabolism of carbohydrates, lipids and proteins, and synthesis of RNA and DNA can retard cell growth and division. The third trimester is the time of rapid brain growth and neurophysiologic organization. High blood alcohol concentrations during this period may impair central nervous system growth and development and limit future intellectual and behavioral capacities.

The role of the timing of exposure has been clearly demonstrated experimentally. In the mouse, abnormalities occurred in the developing brain when high doses of alcohol (350–500 mg/100 ml) were administered on day 7[54]. High ethanol concentrations on day 8 were associated with maxillary hypoplasia and on days 9, 10, and 11 with skeletal anomalies. Similarly, mid-facial abnormalities occurred only when high doses of alcohol were administered within a four hour period on day 7[55].

Rats and mice exposed to high doses of ethanol in week three (late gestation) experienced growth retardation similar to that caused by alcohol exposure throughout pregnancy[37,56]. When alcohol exposure was limited to early pregnancy, there was no significant reduction in birthweight.

Genetic Susceptibility

Susceptibility to alcohol's effects on growth and morphology depends, in part, on genotype. An early mouse model of FAS demonstrated that the strain with lower ADH activity was more sensitive to ethanol than the strain with the greater metabolic capacity[32]. Decreased birthweights were observed among DBA mice but not among C57BL mice given similar doses[57]. Human variability in genetic vulnerability was observed in fraternal twins born to a woman who had consumed at least one quart of red wine and an unspecified amount of hard liquor daily throughout pregnancy[58]. Although both children

135

showed facial characteristics of FAS and were jittery, growth parameters in one were more markedly affected; weight, length and head circumference were at or below the 10th percentile. The weight of the other twin was at the 30th percentile, length at the 15th percentile, and head circumference at the 60th percentile. There are additional reports of fraternal twins in which one was more severely affected[59].

Paternal Drinking

Since most women who drink heavily mate with men who drink heavily, the role of paternal drinking as a mediating factor must be considered. Chronic alcohol consumption in the male disrupts spermatogenesis and reduces the likelihood of fertilization[60]. To date, studies of the association between paternal alcohol consumption and adverse pregnancy outcome have been limited. There has been one report of an association between father's drinking prior to conception and decreased infant birthweight[61]. The mechanisms which underlie this finding remain obscure and further study is required. Experimental findings on the effects of paternal drinking on fetal development have shown increased resorption of defective fetuses and small litter size in rats[62]. In humans, the analogous phenomenon would be an increased tendency for spontaneous abortions. Morphologic abnormalities were not observed in the mouse offspring of alcohol-exposed males[63].

PREVENTION

Clinical Research

At Boston City Hospital (BCH), from 1974 to 1979, all women who spoke English were asked to participate voluntarily in a 15 minute interview survey at the time of registration for prenatal care[64]. Information was gathered about alcohol use, nutrition, smoking patterns, other drug use, socio-economic status, and pregnancy history. Individual questions were asked for consumption of beer, wine, and whiskey. Information on the quantity, frequency and variability of the use of each beverage was recorded, and cumulative score tabulated. Responses were standardized so that a 'drink' was the volume of beverage containing 15 g (0.5 oz) absolute alcohol, e.g. 12 oz of 4% beer, 4 oz of 12% wine, or 1.2 oz of 80 proof liquor. While a structured format was utilized, interviewers encouraged women to elaborate when relevant.

On the basis of self-reports, women were classified as rare, moderate or heavy drinkers. Heavy drinkers consumed at least five drinks on some occasions and 45 drinks per month. Women who drank more than once a month but did not meet the criteria for heavy drinking were classified as moderate drinkers. Rare drinkers either abstained or used alcohol less than once a month and never consumed five drinks on any occasion.

At registration for prenatal care, 9% ($n = 162$) reported drinking heavily. Moderate drinking was reported by 37% ($n = 633$) and 53% ($n = 916$) drank rarely or not at all. The heavy drinkers consumed quantities of alcohol considerably exceeding the minimal criteria for inclusion in this category: reported daily mean was six ounces absolute alcohol (approximately 12 drinks). This was 15 times higher than the amount reported by the moderate drinkers.

The group of women who drank heavily differed from other prenatal patients on a series of behavioral and demographic characteristics. Heavy alcohol consumption was associated with use of cigarettes and other drugs such as marijuana, heroin, barbiturates, psychedelics, and amphetamines. In addition, heavily drinking women were more apt to be exposed to social stress. More were widowed, divorced, or living alone. They reported alcohol-related problems among the men with whom they associated. The women were older and of higher parity. There were no differences in their desire to have a healthy baby, registration for prenatal care before the 26th week, or dietary intake.

Women who reported drinking heavily were encouraged to meet with the project psychiatrist and/or counselor in the prenatal clinic at the time of their scheduled obstetrical appointments[65]. They were informed that they had a better chance of having a healthy baby if they abstained from alcohol use for the duration of their pregnancy. Two-thirds of the women who participated in counseling sessions were considered to have reduced alcohol consumption before the third trimester. Heavily drinking women for whom there was no additional information were grouped according to their responses during the interview at the time of registration.

Complete physical and neurologic evaluations were conducted with 791 infants whose mothers had participated in the prenatal survey[8]. Neonatal examinations were conducted by pediatricians who did not have information about maternal drinking or any other characteristics of the mother, the pregnancy, or the delivery. Infants who were at or below the tenth percentile in weight, length or head circumference were considered to be growth retarded. Any infant with at least three minor or one major abnormality was rated as abnormal. Diagnosis of FAS was restricted to infants who showed signs in each of three categories: growth retardation, CNS anomalies and facial dysmorphology.

Growth retardation occurred among infants born to the women who drank heavily throughout pregnancy significantly more frequently than among children born to the rare and moderate drinkers (Figure 10.1). No significant difference was found between children born to moderate drinkers as compared with those born to women who drank rarely. Neonates born to women who drank heavily early in pregnancy and reduced consumption before the third trimester were comparable to those born to rare and moderate drinkers. Similar findings were observed in the incidence of length and head circumference below the tenth percentile. Abnormalities were identified more frequently among children born to women who continued drinking heavily. These associations were independent of the eight variables thought to influence fetal growth and development: maternal age, parity, ethnicity, cigarette smoking, marijuana use, prepregnancy weight, baby's sex and gestational age.

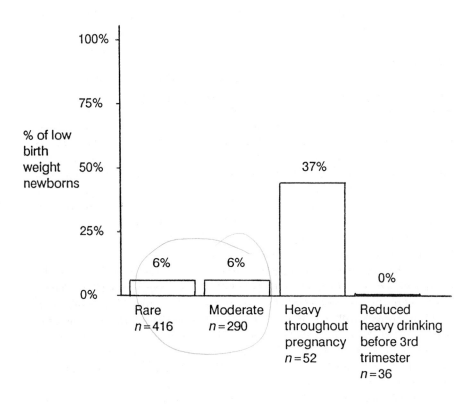

Figure 10.1 Growth retardation and maternal drinking patterns

FAS was diagnosed in five children; one was recognized in neonatal examination and four in follow-up examinations. All five children were born to women who continued to drink heavily throughout pregnancy.

A replication of the Boston City Hospital study was conducted in 1979 at four maternal Health Centers in Stockholm among 464 women[66]. Drinking patterns were identified at time of registration and supportive couseling for problem drinking was integrated with routine prenatal care. The possibility of preventing fetal damage by reducing alcohol consumption was described to all participants. With support from a social worker and nurse, 100% of the women who drank between 3 and 12 drinks a day reduced consumption. Women who drank more than 12 drinks a day were offered intensive counseling; 78% reported that they reduced alcohol intake.

In neonatal examinations conducted with 399 infants, special emphasis was placed on neurological and developmental assessment and on characteristics of FAS. There were no statistically significant differences in growth parameters of infants classified by maternal drinking patterns. More infants of heavy drinkers were placed in the intensive care nursery than those born to light drinkers or abstainers (33% vs. 12%). Two babies were born to women who continued to drink heavily; both were growth-retarded and one was diagnosed as having FAS.

Reduction of heavy drinking has been associated with improved neonatal outcomes on growth parameters, somatic status, and/or CNS development in additional case reports and prospective studies[14,41,67,68]. In a program in Seattle, 80% of the women who drank heavily were able to modify their drinking patterns[67]. Benefits among their children were described as 'dramatic'. Fetal alcohol effects occurred three times more often when mothers continued drinking than when mothers reduced drinking. The Atlanta program reported that 35% of the at-risk women stopped drinking heavily[68]. Increased neurobehavioral alterations were found in infants of women who continued to drink during pregnancy as compared with abstainers and with women who discontinued use by mid-pregnancy[69]. The observed benefits were attributed to cessation of drinking and not to maternal characteristics. The group of women who successfully abstained and the group who failed to respond to treatment were similar on demographic characteristics[64,68]. No significant differences were found in patterns of alcohol consumption reported at the time of clinic registration. Among the women in the Atlanta study, there were no differences in the prevalence of alcohol-related pathology, although the group which continued to drink had begun drinking at an earlier age and were more likely to meet criteria for the diagnosis of alcohol dependence.

Benefits have been observed in older children as well as in neonates. Follow-up examinations were conducted with 74 children from the Stockholm infant study and six additional children whose mothers were abusive drinkers[70]. The median age at the time of follow-up was 22 months (range 18–27 months). Children of alcohol abusers had had the highest incidence of growth retardation, mental retardation, behavioral disturbances and morphologic abnormalities. The postnatal environment did not compensate for these alcohol-related birth defects. In contrast, children of women who reduced consumption did not differ from controls in physical development or behavior. They did, however, display delays in speech.

Evaluations of another group of mother–infant pairs in Sweden demonstrated that five children whose alcohol abusing mothers had stopped drinking in the twelfth gestational week exhibited normal growth, somatic status, and cognitive function at 10 and at 18 months[28]. Subnormal scores were reported among the nine children whose mothers continued heavy drinking throughout pregnancy.

The benefits observed following reduction in alcohol consumption are consistent with the hypothesis that the complete FAS represents the cumulative result of adverse effects throughout gestation. Exposure at critical developmental stages will affect particular systems. When heavy drinking ceases, abnormalities and growth retardation that develop in later stages will be prevented. In addition, maternal capacity to nurture improves when drinking stops.

Experimental studies suggest that an opportunity exists for physiologic restitution and modification of abnormalities which develop secondary to impaired growth[34]. Abnormal embryogenesis, apparent on day 9 in rats exposed to high doses of alcohol on gestational days 5–8, was not apparent on day 20. Similarly, the incidence of defects was much lower in rats exposed to acetaldehyde when examination occurred on the twelfth day rather than on the tenth, with no difference in resorption rates[71,72].

The alterations in neonatal brain size and structure may not be permanent. Cerebellar Purkinje cells revealed significantly smaller nuclei on day 7 among rat pups exposed to alcohol *in utero*[73]. At days 12 and 17 there were no differences, suggesting that alcohol caused a developmental delay with a potential for recovery. Delays in cortical development were also observed[74]. Complete cortical lamination was apparent in controls at 14 days, but not in the alcohol-exposed pups. At 23 days, complete cortical lamination was observed in the alcohol exposed pups.

The capacity for recovery is variable. In mice, cell necrosis affecting the neuroepithelium both in the closed caudal portion of the neural tube and in the unclosed cranial neural tube was observed six hours after ethanol exposure[75]. At 24 hours post-exposure, the neuroepithelium was completely clear of debris resulting from cell necrosis, although some embryos had open neural tube defects and some had been resorbed. Many fetuses survived to day 19 with no apparent gross defects.

While these studies suggest that there is considerable capacity for compensatory growth and repair, further study is required to evaluate functional effects of developmental delays. Alcohol-exposed brains may not be similar to controls on all neurologic, physiologic or behavioral measures.

Clinicians's Role

Greater understanding of the mechanisms of alcohol's effects on fetal development has put new demands on prenatal care providers. Identification and treatment of problem drinking women represents an important challenge for the prevention of alcohol-related birth defects[76]. Since alcohol has the capacity to adversely affect each stage of fetal development, the earlier in pregnancy that heavy drinking ceases, the greater is the potential for improved outcome.

Inclusion of a drinking history as part of every initial evaluation significantly increases recognition of problem drinking. Based on clinical observations, one or two pregnant women a year were considered to be drinking at levels which placed them at risk[20,64,66]. Systematic inquiry revealed that at least 10% of the women were drinking heavily.

Recognition based on stereotypical ideas of the chronic alcoholic is ineffective. Pregnant women usually do not fit the stereotype of the alcoholic since they are young and in the early stages of the disease. Although women who drink heavily differ statistically from other pregnant women on a series of behavioral and demographic traits, these traits have low predictive power and are not effective as specific clinical markers[64]. Blood and breath analyses only reflect recent consumption. Measurement of alcohol content in sweat and urine is not clinically useful. No direct measurements are currently available that will detect alcohol abuse before there is impairment of hepatic or hematopoietic function.

A brief Ten Question Drinking History (TQDH) was developed and incorporated into the Boston City Hospital prenatal clinic record to be administered routinely as part of every intake examination (Table 10.2)[77]. It was demonstrated to be reliable: drinking histories obtained by obstetrical staff using the TQDH with 171 women were comparable to those obtained in a more elaborate research interview. The reliability of the questionnaire was further tested by Larsson[66] who reported good agreement between two occasions of history taking.

Separate, direct questions are asked about the frequency, quantity, and variability of the consumption of beer, wine, and liquor. Validity of self-reports has been shown to improve when specific questions are asked about each beverage[78]. Inquiry about quantity, frequency, and variability of use further improves the accuracy of self-reports. The first nine questions ascertain present drinking projections. The tenth question explores changes in drinking habits during the past year. This allows for discussion of previous patterns, which often provides validation of reports of current use.

Table 10.2 Ten question drinking history

Beer:	How many times per week?
	How many cans each time?
	Ever drink more?
Wine:	How many times per week?
	How many glasses each time?
	Ever drink more?
Liquor:	How many times per week?
	How many drinks each time?
	Ever drink more?

Has your drinking habit changed during the past year?

When the ten questions are asked in a direct, non-judgemental fashion, most patients will accept the clinician's concern and respond honestly. Simple introductory statements reassure the pregnant woman that the questions are being asked in an effort to improve pregnancy outcome. Patients who answer evasively should be calmly and firmly engaged in further discussion. Defensive reactions often indicate alcohol problems.

Administering the TQDH requires less than five minutes when women are not drinking at risk levels. For women who are abusing alcohol, the questionnaire provides a basis for discussing alcohol use and initiating supportive counseling.

Therapy for Women at Risk

Supportive counseling, directed toward attaining and sustaining abstinence, should be initiated as soon as heavy drinking is identified. Maternal concern for the well-being of the child can be a powerful force to engage the pregnant woman in therapy. Pregnancy is a normal crisis in every woman's life with changes in physiology, body image and social role. The sense of responsibility for another life increases receptivity toward assistance from health professionals. Women will respond positively to a hopeful message of potential benefits from reduction (Table 10.3). Provocation of guilt and

142

self-criticism by focusing on damage that may already have been incurred is intolerable and may lead to increased alcohol consumption.

Table 10.3 Accentuate the positive – avoid the negative

POSITIVE	NEGATIVE
'If you stop drinking you have a better chance of having a healthy baby'	'Your drinking has already damaged your baby'
'Your concern for your baby will help you be a good mother'	'If you really loved your baby you would not drink so much'
'You will feel better when you are sober and so will your child'	'Continued drinking will ruin your health and prevent your child from developing normally'

In the program at Boston City Hospital, evaluation of treatment needs began with an assessment of the woman's strengths, including her style of coping with anxiety and depression, her capacity to sustain close relationships with others, her resourcefulness in times of adversity, as well as a specific and detailed history of patterns of substance abuse[65].

A three-phase classification of problem drinking was useful in designing treatment strategies. Classification was based on motivating factors rather than on quantity or duration of use. The phases are not necessarily progressive, although some women had moved from one to the next.

Social problem drinking

For women in this phase, consumption of alcohol was an essential ingredient in their marriages and friendships as well as in the social lives of their communities. They experienced pressure from friends and relatives to continue to drink. Feeling lonely and bored, some used alcohol to gain the illusion of rapid passage of time. Many were able to stop drinking for the duration of pregnancy on the basis of brief supportive counseling with information that they had a better chance of having a healthy child if they abstained. Support and referral to appropriate agencies and self-help groups were most important.

Symptom problem drinking

In this phase, women used drinking to relieve a range of psychological symptoms and depended on alcohol to alter mood and perception. Some sought relief from depression; others used alcohol to blur their awareness of fear, confusion, and discouragement. For many, the added physical and social responsibilities of pregnancy caused ambivalent feelings toward motherhood. Realistic discussion of conflicts about their roles as mothers helped reduce feelings of inadequacy. They needed repetition of information about pregnancy and the birth process that had been presented by other staff members. Women in this group required extensive counseling and support with a variety of social problems as well as with the normal crises secondary to pregnancy.

Alcohol dependence (alcoholism)

Women in this phase had a physiological tolerance for and a dependency on alcohol and met criteria for the diagnosis of alcoholism. Most were consuming between one half to one quart of liquor a day or its equivalent. Several had medical complications secondary to alcohol use, including hepatitis, pancreatitis, and non-diabetic ketoacidosis. In addition to their medical needs, they required extensive assistance with child care and social service problems. Alcoholism treatment centers, halfway houses, and AA groups were required to provide therapy and support.

Therapeutic intervention in all phases of problem drinking is facilitated by an alliance between the woman and the therapist, focused on having a healthy child. Pregnant women establish sustained relationships with health professionals in which medical rather than moralistic values predominate. When providers express optimism, patients feel more able to master the problem. They respond readily to therapy integrated with routine care.

Heavy drinking is often associated with a continuum of prenatal risk factors including smoking, malnutrition, stress and other drug use. Participation in a program focused on reduction of alcohol use facilitates discussion of other life style issues and encourages utilization of other health and social service agencies.

CONCLUSION

Ethanol has the potential to cause a greater variety of metabolic and physiologic disturbances of fetal development than any other commonly ingested substance. The clinical and experimental literature provides an ever-increasing understanding of the mechanisms underlying alcohol's adverse effects on fetal development. Effects vary with each gestational stage. Alcohol consumption throughout pregnancy is associated with the most severe outcome. The demonstrated benefits when heavy drinking ceases reinforces the value of providing supportive therapy to women at risk. The prenatal setting is an important site for prevention of alcohol-related birth defects. Identification and treatment of problem drinking pregnant women holds the greatest promise for the prevention of alcohol-related birth defects.

REFERENCES

1. Warner, R.H. and Rosett, H.L. (1975). The effects of drinking on offspring: an historical survey of the American and British literature. *J. Stud. Alcohol.*, **36**, 1395–420
2. Burton, R. (1906). [Orig. 1621]. *The Anatomy of Melancholy*. Vol. 1, Part I, Section 2: Causes of melancholy. (London: William Tegg)
3. Lemoine, P., Harousseau, H., Borteyru, J-P. and Menuet, J-C. (1968). Les enfants de parents alcooliques: anomalies observees a propos de 127 cas. (Children of alcoholic parents: anomalies observed in 127 cases.) *Quest. Med.*, **21**, 476–82
4. Jones, K.L. and Smith, D.W. (1973). Recognition of the fetal alcohol syndrome in early infancy. *Lancet*, **2**, 999–1001
5. Rosett, H.L. and Weiner, L. (1984). *Alcohol and the Fetus: A Clinical Perspective.* (New York: Oxford University Press)
6. Rosett, H.L. (1980). A clinical perspective of the fetal alcohol syndrome. *Alcoholism Clin. Exp. Res.*, **4**, 119–22
7. Hill, R.M. (1976). Fetal malformations and antiepileptic drugs. *Am. J. Dis. Child.*, **130**, 923–5
8. Rosett, H.L., Weiner, L., Lee, A., Zuckerman, B., Dooling, E. and Oppenheimer, E. (1983). Patterns of alcohol consumption and fetal development. *Obstet. Gynecol.*, **61**, 539–46
9. Dehaene, P., Walbaum, R., Titran, M., Samaille-Villette, C., Samaille, P., Crepin, G., Delahousse, G., Decocq, J., Delcroix, M., Caquant, F. and Querleu, D. (1977). La descendance des meres alcooliques chroniques: a propos de 16 cas d'alcoolisme foetal. (The offspring of alcoholic mothers: a report of 16 cases of fetal alcohol syndrome.) *Rev. Franc. Gynecol. Obstet.*, **72**, 491–8
10. Jones, K.L., Smith, D.W., Ulleland, C.N. and Streissguth, A.P. (1973). Pattern of malformation in offspring of chronic alcoholic mothers. *Lancet*, **1**, 1267–71
11. Sokol, R.J. (1981). Alcohol and abnormal outcomes of pregnancy. *Can. Med. Assoc. J.*, **125**, 143–8
12. May, P.A. and Hymbaugh, K.J. (1982/83). A pilot project on fetal alcohol syndrome among American Indians. *Alcohol Health Res. World*, **7**, 3–9
13. Abel, E.L. and Sokol, R.J. (1987). Incidence of fetal alcohol syndrome and economic impact of FAS-related anomalies. *Drug Alcohol Depend.*, **19**, 51–70
14. Olegard, R., Sabel, K-G., Aronsson, M., Sandin, B., Johansson, P.R., Carlsson, C., Kyllerman, M., Iverson, K. and Hrbek, A. (1979). Effects on the child of alcohol abuse during pregnancy: retrospective and prospective studies. *Acta Paediatr. Scand. (Suppl.)*, **275**, 112–21

15. Clarren, S.K. and Smith, D.W. (1978). The fetal alcohol syndrome. *N. Engl. J. Med.*, **298**, 1063-7
16. Streissguth, A.P. and LaDue, R.A. (1987). Fetal alcohol: teratogenic causes of developmental disabilities. In Schroeder, S.R. (ed.) *Toxic Substances and Mental Retardation*, pp.1-32 (Boston: American Association of Mental Deficiency, Monograph #8)
17. Frias, J.L., Wilson, A.L. and King, G.J. (1982). A cephalometric study of fetal alcohol syndrome. *J. Pediatr.*, **101**, 870-3
18. Ouellette, E.M., Rosett, H.L., Rosman, N.P. and Weiner, L. (1977). The adverse effects on offspring of maternal alcohol abuse during pregnancy. *N. Engl. J. Med.*, **297**, 528-30
19. Hanson, J.W., Streissguth, A.P. and Smith, D.W. (1978). The effects of moderate alcohol consumption during pregnancy on fetal growth and morphogenesis. *J. Pediatr.*, **92**, 457-60
20. Sokol, R.J., Miller, S.I. and Reed, G. (1980). Alcohol abuse during pregnancy: an epidemiological model. *Alcoholism Clin. Exp. Res.*, **4**, 135-45
21. Abel, E.L. (1984). *Fetal Alcohol Syndrome and Fetal Alcohol Effects*. (New York: Plenum Press)
22. Majewski, F. (1981). Alcohol embryopathy: some facts and speculations about pathogenesis. *Neurobehav. Toxicol. Teratol.*, **3**, 129-44
23. Spohr, H.L. and Steinhausen, H.C. (1984). Clinical psychopathological and developmental aspects in children with the fetal alcohol syndrome: a four-year follow-up study. In *CIBA Foundation Symposium 105, Mechanisms of Alcohol Damage in Utero*, pp. 197-217. (London: Pitman Press)
24. Streissguth, A.P., Barr, H.M. and Marin, D.C. (1984). Alcohol exposure in utero and functional deficits in children during the first four years of life. In *CIBA Foundation Symposium 105, Mechanisms of Alcohol Damage in Utero*, pp. 176-96. (London: Pitman Press)
25. Bierich, J.R. (1978). Pranatale schadigungen durch alkohol. (Prenatal damage from alcohol.) *Der Internist.*, **19**, 131-9
26. Koranyi, G. and Csiky, E. (1978). Az embryopathia alcoholica gyermekkroban eszlelheto tuneteirol. (Signs of alcohol embryopathy apparent in childhood.) *Orvosi Hetilap.*, **119**, 2923-9
27. Nanson, J., Habbick, B.F., Casey, R.E. and Zaleski, W.A. (1981). Fetal alcohol syndrome in Saskatchewan: some preliminary findings. *Perinatal Bull.*, **14**, 3-4
28. Aronson, M. and Olegard, R. (1985). Fetal alcohol effects in pediatrics and child psychology. In Rydberg, U., Alling, C., Engel, J., Pernow, B., Pellborn, L.A. and Rossner, S. (eds.) *Alcohol and the Developing Brain*, pp. 135-45. (New York: Raven Press)
29. Fisher, S.E., Atkinson, M., Burnap, J.K., Jacobson, S., Sehgal, P.K., Scott, W. and Van Thil, D.V. (1982). Ethanol-associated selective fetal malnutrition: a contributing factor in the fetal alcohol syndrome. *Alcoholism Clin. Exp. Res.*, **6**, 197-201
30. Pratt, O.E. (1980). The fetal alcohol syndrome: transport of nutrients and transfer of alcohol and acetaldehyde from mother to fetus. In Sandler, M. (ed.) *Psychopharmacology of Alcohol*, pp. 229-56. (New York: Raven Press)
31. Ellis, F.W. and Pick, J.R. (1980). An animal model of the fetal alcohol syndrome in beagles. *Alcoholism Clin. Exp. Res.*, **4**, 123-34
32. Chernoff, G.F. (1977). The fetal alcohol syndrome in mice: an animal model. *Teratology*, **15**, 223-30
33. Randall, C.L. and Taylor, W.J. (1979). Prenatal ethanol exposure in mice: teratogenic effects. *Teratology*, **19**, 302-12
34. Anders, K. and Persaud, T.V.N. (1980). Compensatory embryonic development in the rat following maternal treatment with ethanol. *Anat. Anaz.*, **148**, 375-83
35. Skosyreva, A.M. (1973). Vliyaniye etilovogo spirta na razvitiye embrionov stadii organogeneza. (Effect of ethyl alcohol on embryo development at the stage of organogenesis.) *Akush. Ginekol. (Moskow)*, **4**, 15-8
36. Abel, E.L. (1978). Effects of ethanol on pregnant rats and their offspring. *Psychopharmacology*, **57**, 5-11
37. Abel, E.L. (1979). Prenatal effects of alcohol on adult learning in rat. *Pharmacol. Biochem. Behav.*, **10**, 239-43

38. Samson, H.H. and Grant, K.A. (1984). Ethanol induced microcephaly in the neonatal rat: relation to dose. *Alcoholism Clin. Exp. Res.*, **8**, 201–3
39. Pierce, D.R. and West, J.R. (1986). Blood alcohol concentration: a critical factor for producing fetal alcohol effects. *Alcohol*, **3**, 269–72
40. Kaminiski, M., Franc, M., Lebouvier, M., duMazaubrun, C. and Rumeau-Rouquette, C. (1981). Moderate alcohol use and pregnancy outcome. *Neurobehav. Toxicol. Teratol.*, **3**, 173–81
41. Seidenberg, J. and Majewski, F. (1978). Zur Haeufigkeit der Alkoholembryopathie in den Verschiedenen Phasen der muetterlichen Alkoholkrankheit. (Frequency of alcohol embryopathy in the different stages of maternal alcoholism.) *Hamburg Suchtgefahren*, **24**, 63–75
42. Kuzma, J.W. and Sokol, R.J. (1982). Maternal drinking behavior and decreased intra-uterine growth. *Alcoholism Clin. Exp. Res.*, **6**, 396–402
43. Silva, V.A., Laranjeira, R.R., Dolnikoff, M., Grinfeld, H. and Masur, J. (1981). Alcohol consumption during pregnancy and newborn outcome: a study in Brazil. *Neurobehav. Toxicol. Teratol.*, **3**, 169–72
44. Little, R.E. (1977). Moderate alcohol use during pregnancy and decreased infant birth weight. *Am. J. Public Health*, **67**, 1154–6
45. Mills, J.L., Graubard, B.I., Harley, E.E., Rhoads, G.G. and Berendes, H.W. (1984). Maternal alcohol consumption and birth weight. *J. Am. Med. Assoc.*, **252**, 1875–9
46. Tennes, K. and Blackard, C. (1980). Maternal alcohol consumption, birth weight and minor physical anomalies. *Am. J. Obstet. Gynecol.*, **138**, 774–80
47. Hingson, R., Alpert, J.J., Day, N., Dooling, E., Kayne, H., Morelock, S., Oppenheimer, E. and Zuckerman, B. (1982). Effects of maternal drinking and marijuana use on fetal growth and development. *Pediatrics*, **70**, 539–46
48. Marbury, M.C., Linn, S., Monson, R.R., Schoenbaum, S.C., Stubblefield, P.G. and Ryan, K.J. (1983). The association of alcohol consumption with outcome of pregnancy. *Am. J. Public Health*, **73**, 1165–8
49. Lumley, J., Correy, J.F., Newman, N.M. and Curran, J.T. (1985). Cigarette smoking, alcohol consumption and fetal outcome in Tasmania. *Aust. N.Z. J. Obstet. Gynaecol.*, **25**, 33–5
50. Ernhart, C.B., Sokol, R.J., Martier, S., Morton, P., Nadler, D., Ager, J.W. and Wolf, A. (1987). Alcohol teratogenicity in the human: a detailed assessment of specificity, critical period, and threshold. *Am. J. Obstet. Gynecol.*, **156**, 33–9
51. USDHHS (1987). *Alcohol and Health, Sixth Special Report to the U.S. Congress.* (Washington, DC: U.S. Government Printing Office)
52. Clarren, S.K. (1982). The diagnosis and treatment of fetal alcohol syndrome. *Comp. Therapy*, **8**, 41–6
53. Jellinek, E.M. (1960). *The Disease Concept of Alcoholism*, pp. 36–40. (New Haven: New College University Press)
54. Webster, W.S., Walsh, D.A., Lipson, A.H. and McEwan, S.E. (1980). Teratogenesis after acute alcohol exposure in inbred and outbred mice. *Neurobehav. Toxicol.*, **2**, 227–34
55. Sulik, K.K. and Johnston, M.C. (1983). Sequence of developmental alterations following acute ethanol exposure in mice: craniofacial features of the fetal alcohol syndrome. *Am. J. Anat.*, **166**, 257–69
56. Lochry, E.A., Randall, C.L., Goldsmith, A.A. and Sutker, P.B. (1982). Effects of acute alcohol exposure during selected days of gestation in C3H mice. *Neurobehav. Toxicol. Teratol.*, **4**, 15–9
57. Yanai, J. and Ginsburg, B.E. (1977). A developmental study of ethanol effect on behavior and physical dependence in mice. *Alcoholism Clin. Exp. Res.*, **1**, 325–33
58. Christoffel, K.K. and Salafsky, I. (1957). Fetal alcohol syndrome in dizygotic twins. *J. Pediatr.*, **87**, 963–7
59. Santolaya, J.M., Martinez, G., Gorostiza, E., Aizpiri, J. and Hernandez, M. (1978). Alcoholism fetal (Fetal alcohol syndrome). *Drogalcohol.*, **3**, 183–92
60. Van Thiel, D.H. and Gavaler, J.S. (1982). The adverse effects of ethanol upon hypothalamic–pituitary–gonadal function in males and females compared and contrasted. *Alcoholism Clin. Exp. Res.*, **6**, 179–85

147

61. Little, R.E. and Sing, C.S. (1987). Father's drinking and infant birth weight: report on an association. *Teratology*, **36**, 59–65
62. Anderson, R.A., Beyler, S.A. and Zaneveld, L.J.D. (1978). Alterations of male reproduction induced by chronic ingestion of ethanol: development of an animal model. *Fertil. Steril.*, **30**, 103–5
63. Randall, C.L., Burling, T.A., Lochry, E.A. and Sutker, P.B. (1982). The effect of paternal alcohol consumption on fetal development in mice. *Drug Alcohol Depend.*, **9**, 89–95
64. Weiner, L., Rosett, H.L., Edelin, K.C., Alpert, J.J. and Zuckerman, B. (1983). Alcohol consumption by pregnant women. *Obstet. Gynecol.*, **61**, 6–12
65. Rosett, H.L., Weiner, L. and Edelin, K.C. (1983). Treatment experience with pregnant problem drinkers. *J. Am. Med. Assoc.*, **249**, 2029–33
66. Larrson, G. (1983). Prevention of fetal alcohol effects: an antenatal program for early detection of pregnancies at risk. *Acta Obstet. Gynecol. Scand.*, **62**, 171–8
67. Little, R.E., Young, A., Streissguth, A.P. and Uhl, C.N. (1984). Preventing fetal alcohol effects: effectiveness of a demonstration project. In *CIBA Foundation Symposium 105, Mechanisms of Alcohol Damage in Utero*, pp. 254–74. (London: Pitman Press)
68. Smith, I.E., Lancaster, J.S., Moss-Wells, S., Coles, C.D. and Falek, A. (1987). Identifying high-risk pregnant drinkers: biological and behavioral correlates of continuous heavy drinking during pregnancy. *J. Stud. Alcohol.*, **48**, 304–9
69. Coles, C.D., Smith, I.E., Fernhoff, P.M. and Falek, A. (1985). Neonatal neurobehavioral characteristics as correlates of maternal alcohol use during gestation. *Alcoholism Clin. Exp. Res.*, **9**, 454–60
70. Larrson, G., Bohlin, A-B. and Tunnell, R. (1985). Prospective study of children exposed to variable amounts of alcohol in utero. *Arch. Dis. Child.*, **60**, 316–21
71. O'Shea, K.S. and Kaufman, M.H. (1981). Effect of acetaldehyde on the neuroepithelium of early mouse embryos. *J. Anat.*, **132**, 107–18
72. Dreosti, I.E., Ballard, F.J., Belling, G.B., Record, I.R., Manuel, S.J. and Hertzel, B.S. (1981). The effect of ethanol and acetaldehyde on DNA synthesis in growing cells and on fetal development in the rat. *Alcoholism Clin. Exp. Res.*, **5**, 357–62
73. Volk, B., Maletz, J., Tiedemann, M., Mall, G., Kleun, C. and Berlet, H.H. (1981). Impaired maturation of Purkinje cells in the fetal alcohol syndrome of the rat: light and electron microscopic investigations. *Acta Neuropathol.*, **54**, 19–29
74. Jacobson, S., Rich, J. and Tovsky, N.J. (1978). Delayed myelination and lamination in the cerebral cortex of the albino rat as a result of the fetal alcohol syndrome. In Galanter, M. (ed.) *Currents in Alcoholism*, Vol. 5, pp. 123–33. (New York: Grune and Stratton)
75. Bannigan, J. and Burke, P. (1982). Ethanol teratogenicity in mice: a light microscopic study. *Teratology*, **26**, 247–54
76. Weiner, L., Morse, B.A. and Garrido, P. (1988). FAS/FAE: Focusing prevention on women at risk. *Int. J. Addict.*, (in press)
77. Weiner, L., Rosett, H.L. and Edelin, K.C. (1982). Behavioral evaluation of fetal alcohol education for physicians. *Alcoholism Clin. Exp. Res.*, **6**, 230–3
78. Cahalan, D., Cissin, I.R. and Crossley, H.M. (1969). *American Drinking Practices*. (New Brunswick, New Jersey: Rutgers Center of Alcohol Studies)

11

Breastfeeding by the Chemically Dependent Woman

Jeanne M Wilton

INTRODUCTION

Approximately 60% of women in the USA now breastfeed at hospital discharge[1]. Most of these women, however, are in middle- to upper-income brackets. The breastfeeding rate is much lower (20–30%) in lower socioeconomic groups[2].

Breastfeeding is advantageous to any mother–baby dyad: more easily digestible nutrients for the baby, antibodies to fight infection, bonding, convenience, and more rapid uterine involution for the mother. These advantages are even more likely to assist the mother who was chemically dependent during pregnancy. The calming effect that prolactin has on the brain during suckling may help the mother deal with a baby who may be jittery. During breastfeeding the baby must be held close for long periods of time which may be soothing to the baby's irritable behavior. If the mother bottle feeds she should be counseled to try to duplicate this swaddling. The feeling that she is providing total nutrition for this baby may increase her self-esteem and decrease her dependency on health care providers. However, it is important that she remain chemically free and be followed closely to monitor her progress. Promoting breastfeeding for these women is therefore important if they meet criteria of being motivated, chemically free at the time of delivery or under appropriate maintenance therapy (such as methadone).

Most medication a mother ingests during lactation is passed through her breastmilk. The concentration of that drug in the breastmilk, however, depends on many factors which include the solubility of the drug, the protein binding of the drug and the pH of the drug. The time of ingestion by the mother, age of the baby, as well as possible cumulative effects over time will also affect whether a drug can be recommended. For this reason the infant of a chemically dependent woman is at much higher risk with the use of certain

149

medications. The following is a summary of the latest findings on the most commonly abused drugs. Some of these are necessary for psychiatric use and in controlled doses may be acceptable, but most when abused can be harmful to the baby.

NARCOTIC ANALGESICS

Most narcotic analgesics in therapeutic doses pose no problem in breastfed babies, but with regular use can cause symptoms of dependence and withdrawal. Morphine and opium derivatives are probably the most studied. In single doses a minimal effect is seen but with prolonged use, particularly with heroin habituation, withdrawal symptoms can occur[3-5] (Table 11.1). Significant amounts of heroin are found in breastmilk, and most authorities believe this drug should be avoided[5,9]. Codeine has not been detected in breastmilk but may accumulate, and signs of neonatal depression can be observed[5]. Babies whose mothers have used Darvon and Percodan in round-the-clock doses[5] have shown evidence of failure to thrive and drowsiness . Demerol is present in trace amounts in breastmilk; drowsiness and poor feeding should also be observed for with large doses[5]. Methadone is secreted in small amounts in breastmilk. If the infant is withdrawn, breastfeeding can be continued if the mother is on a low dose (<20 mg/24 h)[4-6]. The infant again should be monitored for depression and symptoms of failure to thrive[5,6] (Table 11.2).

T's and Blue's (pentazocine and tripelennamine) are often replaced for methadone. There is no data on pentazocine and lactation, and the AAP feels tripelennamine is safe[4,9].

AMPHETAMINES

Amphetamines are excreted in breastmilk and may cause stimulation in infants, with jitteriness, irritability and sleeplessness[4,5]. Long-term possible cumulative effects have not been studied.

ANTIPSYCHOTICS

Antipsychotics as well as antidepressants have been studied the most because psychiatrists often must keep pregnant and lactating women on these medications to maintain appropriate therapy. Robinson et al.[7] outline the use of psychotropic drugs very well in their recent article. Haloperidol (Haldol) is not recommended in lactation because the amount excreted in breastmilk is unknown and animal studies have shown serious behavioral abnormalities[7]. Chlorpromazine or other phenothiazines should be used with caution. The amount excreted in breastmilk is less than one third of maternal plasma, but drowsiness, possible prolonged jaundice, and galactorrhea can occur with large doses[4,7,8].

Table 11.1 Drugs that are contraindicated in lactation

Drug	Effect on neonate	Reference
Narcotic analgesics		
Heroin	Can cause prolonged addiction in infants Significant amounts found in milk	3, 4, 5
Anesthetics		
Phencyclidine (PCP)	Increased concentrations in breastmilk, significant activity changes noted in animal research	5, 12, 13
Cocaine	Case report of cocaine intoxication after mother smoked and breastfed – dilated pupils, hypertension, tachycardia, and irritability	14
Antipsychotics		
Haloperidol (Haldol)	Animal studies show serious behavior abnormalities	7
Antidepressants		
Lithium	Concentrated 50% maternal dose in milk, cyanosis, poor muscle tone, ECG changes	5, 7, 8
Antianxiety		
Meprobamate (Equinil/Miltown)	Concentrated in milk 2–4 times	5, 7, 8, 9
Librium	Lethargy, impaired temperature regulation, possible increased incidence of newborn jaundice	7, 8, 9
Diazepam (Valium)	Lethargy, weight loss, failure to thrive, drowsiness	5, 7, 8
Hypnotics		
Marijuana	Produces structural changes in brain cells of laboratory animals; excreted in breastmilk	5, 9

Table 11.2 Drugs which may be used with caution in lactation

Drug	Effect on neonate	Reference
Narcotic analgesics		
Darvon	50% of amount in plasma, large dose can cause failure to feed and drowsiness, small doses – no effect	5
Methadone	Withdraw infant first, if mother on low maintenance, may breastfeed if monitored for evidence of depression and failure to thrive	4, 5, 6
Antidepressants		
Tricyclics (amitryptilline, desipramine)	Small amount excreted in breastmilk, effect on developing neurotransmitter system unknown	7, 8
Antipsychotics		
Chlorpromazine	Small amount excreted may cause prolonged jaundice, drowsiness, galactorrhea	4, 7, 8
Barbiturates		
(phenobarbital, secobarbital, etc.	Drowsiness in high doses; 1 case methemoglobinemia	4, 5, 7
Sedatives, hypnotics		
Alcohol	In large doses (1 – 2 g/kg) causes inhibition of milk-ejection reflex, drowsiness, pseudo-Cushing syndrome reported, abnormal weight gain	5, 6, 7
Chloral hydrate	Drowsiness	4, 5
Stimulants		
Nicotine	Decreased milk production; vomiting, diarrhea, restlessness	5, 15
Amphetamine	Irritability, poor sleeping patterns	4, 5

ANTIDEPRESSANTS

The tricyclic antidepressants (amytryptilline, desipramine) are secreted in small amounts in breastmilk[7,8]. So far there have been no adverse side effects, but caution is advised due to the unknown effect on the neurotransmitter system of the neonate[7] (Table 11.2).

Lithium, however, is contraindicated in the lactating mother[5,7,8]. One-half that in serum is present in breastmilk. Lithium affects amine metabolism and infants have experienced cyanosis, poor muscle tone, and ECG changes[7].

ANTIANXIETY AGENTS

Recently the benzodiazepines (Librium, Valium) have been quoted as contraindicated in lactating mothers[7-9]. Like Lithium, these medications have been listed as being safe by the American Academy of Pediatrics[4]. If these drugs are abused, serious consequences can result in the neonate. An increased incidence of jaundice can occur as well as lethargy and impaired temperature regulation[7,8]. Valium can accumulate with long-term use and weight loss can occur after the third day due to the sedative effect of the medication[5,7,8]. Single doses, however, under 10 mg, may pose no problems[5].

Meprobamate (Equinil/Miltown) is concentrated in milk two to four times and is not recommended in lactation[5,7-9].

BARBITURATES

Barbiturates (Nembutal, Pentobarbital, Phenobarbital) can be used with caution while breastfeeding, although short-acting varieties are preferable[4]. Hypnotic doses (>30 mcg/ml) can cause sedation, decreased weight gain, and decreased responsiveness in the infant[4,5]. If the mother breastfeeds soon after such a dose, decreased sucking is also possible[5]. Phenobarbital has been implicated in one case of methemoglobinemia[4]. Barbiturates can also increase the activity of drug-metabolizing enzymes in the infant's liver, therefore affecting other drugs passed through breastmilk[7].

HYPNOTICS

Hypnotics that can be used with caution while breastfeeding include Doriden and chloral hydrate[4,5]. Both are passed through breastmilk and may cause drowsiness and possible sedation if fed at peak milk concentration[5]. Marijuana has been shown in laboratory animals to produce structural changes in brain cells, impairing DNA and RNA formation[5,9]. It is rapidly excreted into breastmilk where it can remain for a prolonged period[5,9]. At the Perinatal Center for Chemical Dependence, mothers are not allowed to breastfeed if they use marijuana. Methaqualone (Quaalude) has not been studied in breastfeeding, but is not recommended in pregnancy[9].

ANESTHETICS, SEDATIVES

Alcohol, one of the most commonly used drugs, reaches levels in breastmilk that are equivalent to plasma levels[5]. Chronic drinking and breastfeeding has been linked with obesity and pseudo-Cushing syndrome[5,10].

In one report, a baby with pseudo-Cushing syndrome showed an increased rate of weight gain, but decreased growth rate[10]. A thymic shadow was present and symptoms were relieved when the mother stopped drinking. Cobo[11] found that alcohol in quantities of $1-2$ g/kg inhibited the milk-ejection reflex significantly. Therefore, alcohol in moderation may be fairly safe in lactation, but chronic use should be discouraged. At the Perinatal Center for Chemical Dependence, lactating mothers are advised to pump and discard the milk for 24 hours after ingesting large amounts of alcohol.

Phencyclidine (PCP) has been shown to be concentrated in breastmilk[12]. In rat studies significant changes in brain enzymes have been demonstrated, although no studies have been done with humans[12,13].

STIMULANTS

Cocaine is a very commonly abused drug today in the United States. Chasnoff et al.[14] described one case where a mother breastfed her infant while using cocaine over four hours[14]. The infant was admitted to the emergency room suffering from signs of cocaine intoxication – dilated pupils, hypertension, tachycardia, and irritability. Cocaine was still found in the mother's breastmilk 48 hours later. Therefore, the mother who abuses cocaine is advised not to breastfeed or to pump for 72 hours following cocaine use.

Nicotine can be used with caution while breastfeeding. Mothers should know that it is passed through breastmilk, although not in as high a concentration as through the placenta[15].

There has only been one case reported of restlessness and circulatory disturbance in the baby of a heavy smoker, but in general there are no apparent effects on the infant[5]. Smoking has been shown to decrease milk production and may interfere with let-down if smoking occurs right before a feeding[5].

SURVEY

Since very little information is available on the breastfeeding rate of women who are chemically dependent, a brief survey was conducted of 50 patients in the Perinatal Center for Chemical Dependence at Northwestern Memorial Hospital. Demographically, the women in this clinic have an average of 8.4 years of drug abuse, range in age from 19–37 years with an average of 27, are mostly black (57%), single (62%), and on Medicaid (74%). Demographics on this particular surveyed population were not taken.

Immediately postpartum, nine women were asked their selected feeding method, whether they were counseled not to breastfeed, whether they would have breastfed if they were not using drugs, and why they decided to breastfeed. Only two (22%) of these nine women decided to breastfeed and they did so because they had breastfed previous children. None of the respondents were counseled not to breastfeed and none responded that they would have breastfed if not using drugs.

The most common drug of choice prenatally was cocaine (83%). One woman was on methadone maintenance.

Forty-one mothers were polled on their visit to the Perinatal Center for Chemical Dependence Clinic for follow-up postpartum. At delivery, 17% ($n=7$) of these women had stated they were breastfeeding, 78% ($n=32$) bottle feeding, and 5% ($n=2$) feeding with breast and bottle. At the time of follow-up interview, only 5% ($n=2$) of the mothers were still totally breastfeeding, 90% ($n=37$) bottle feeding, and 5% ($n=2$) feeding both breast and bottle. Mothers who discontinued breastfeeding ($n=5$) stopped at age one week, two months, one day, two days, and one did not answer this question. The reasons given for stopping were sore nipples, going back to work, not eating right food and smoking, difficulty grasping nipple, baby 'sucks too hard', and positive HIV antibody. Nineteen (46%) of the mothers stated they were no longer using drugs, 15 (36%) stated they were, and 7 did not answer. Cocaine again was the most common drug of choice postnatally (34%), followed by alcohol (7%).

It was hypothesized by this investigator that this population would breastfeed at a lower rate than the general population and that the reason for stopping would be fussiness or jitteriness in the baby. This brief survey showed that indeed this population does breastfeed at a lower rate than the general population, even compared with studies done on lower socio-economic groups[1,2]. However, reasons for stopping appeared to not be related to fussiness of the infant. Certainly a more precise survey and larger sample size may reveal more significant data.

However this survey does show that some mothers are interested in breastfeeding if drug-free at delivery.

The choice of whether to breast or bottle feed should be discussed prenatally with the women in a chemical dependence program. Other factors besides drug use may affect her decision, such as age, exposure to other mothers who have breastfed, socioeconomic status, and support for the breastfeeding, particularly from the father of the baby. It is not sufficient to ask the mother which method she chooses. She needs to make an informed decision, and the advantages of each feeding method should be clearly discussed with her. If she does decide to breastfeed she should be supported in the decision and counseled on her use of illicit drugs. At the Perinatal Center for Chemical Dependence, the mother must be drug-free for three months during pregnancy, substantiated by urine toxicology, in treatment and consistent with her appointments, HIV negative, and compliant with prenatal recommendations.

Breastfeeding classes prenatally can help her feel more comfortable with her decision. Postpartum she should be followed, counseled and tested frequently for any use of drugs. At Northwestern, alcohol and marijuana use are particularly emphasized since they are common recreational drugs. Support is essential for prolonged duration of breastfeeding. If a hotline or lactation consultant is available, she should be encouraged to call or a direct referral made for close follow-up. These mothers need positive feedback that they can be good mothers. Breastfeeding can help accomplish this when the women see their babies grow and thrive from their own mother's milk. Warm and caring personnel can help accomplish a good breastfeeding relationship for the mother and baby.

A WORD ABOUT AIDS

Due to the recent rise of AIDS and ARC it is important to mention that the HIV antigen has been isolated in breastmilk[16], and there have been cases of suspected AIDS transmission via breastmilk[17]. Therefore, it is recommended that every chemically dependent woman be screened for the HIV antibody and, if positive, be advised not to breastfeed her infant.

SUMMARY

Women who abuse drugs should be counseled not to breastfeed if their addiction is such that the drug will seriously affect the neonate. The necessity of a therapeutic drug must be weighed against the potential effects on the neonate. It also appears that chemically dependent women may not desire to breastfeed as much as the general population, although there is much need for further study in this area.

At the Perinatal Center for Chemical Dependence, women who are drug free for three months at delivery and are highly motivated are encouraged to breastfeed. Breastfeeding is advantageous for these women because it can increase their bonding with a baby who may be irritable and provide them with increased self-esteem when they realize they are providing total nutrition for their infants. With continued support for the breastfeeding relationship and close follow-up, these mothers should be able to breastfeed their infants successfully.

ACKNOWLEDGEMENTS

Great appreciation is given to Pat Shaw, RN and Ira Chasnoff, MD for help on this manuscript.

REFERENCES

1. Martinez, G.A. and Krieger, F.W. (1985). 1984 Milk-feeding patterns in the United States. *Pediatrics*, **76**, 1004–8
2. Rassin, D., Richardson, J., Baranowski, T., Nader, P., Guenther, N., Bee, D. and Brown, J. (1984). Incidence of breastfeeding in a low socioeconomic group of mothers in the United States: Ethnic patterns. *Pediatrics*, **73**, 132–7
3. Cobrink, R.W., Hood, R.T. Jr. and Chasid, E. (1959). The effect of maternal narcotic addiction on the newborn infant: Review of literature and report of 22 cases. *Pediatrics*, **24**, 288
4. Committee on Drugs. (1984). The transfer of drugs and other chemicals into human breast milk. *Perinatal Press*, **8**(5), 67–75
5. Lauwers, J. and Woessner, C. (1983). *Counseling the Nursing Mother*. (New Jersey: Avery Publishing Group, Inc.)
6. Blinick, G., Jerez, E. and Wallach, R.C. (1976). Drug addiction in pregnancy and the neonate. *Am. J. Obstet. Gynecol.*, **125**, 135
7. Robinson, G.E., Steward, D.E. and Flak, E. (April 1986). The rational use of psychotropic drugs in pregnancy and postpartum. *Can. J. Psychol.*, **37**, 183–90
8. Calabrese, J. and Gulledge, A.D. (1985). Psychotropics during pregnancy and lactation: A review. *Psychosomatics*, **26**(5), 413–26
9. Briggs, G., Freeman, K. and Yaffe, S. (1986). *Drugs in Pregnancy and Lactation*, 2nd Edition. (Baltimore: Williams & Wilkins)
10. Binkiewicz, A., Robinson, M.J. and Senior, B. (1978). Pseudo-Cushing syndrome caused by alcohol in breast milk. *J. Pediatr.*, **93**(6), 965–7
11. Cobo, E. (1973). Effect of different doses of ethanol on the milk-ejecting reflex in lactating women. *Am. J. Obstet. Gynecol.*, **113**(6), 817–21
12. Kaufman, K., Petrucha, R., Pitts, F. and Wekkes, M. (1983). PCP in amniotic fluid and breast milk: Case report. *J. Clin. Psychiatr.*, **44**, 269–70
13. Chasnoff, I., Burns, W., Hatcher, R. and Burns, K. (1984). Phencyclidine: Effects on the fetus and neonate. *Devel. Pharmacol. Ther.*, **6**, 404–8
14. Chasnoff, I., Lewis, D.E. and Squires, L. (1987). Cocaine: Intoxication in a breastfed infant. *Pediatrics*, **80**, 836–8
15. Luck, W. and Nau, H. (1984). Exposure to the fetus, neonate, and nursed infant to nicotine and continine from maternal smoking. *N. Engl. J. Med.*, **672**
16. Thiry, L., Sprecher-Goldberger, S., Jonckheer, T., Levy, J., Van de Perre, P., Henrivaux, P., Cogniaux-Leclerc, J. and Clumeck, N. (1985). Isolation of AIDS virus from cell-free breast milk of three healthy virus carriers. *Lancet*, 891–2
17. Boyes, S. (1987). AIDS virus in breast milk: A new threat to neonates and donor breast milk banks. *Neonatal Network*, 37–9

12

Parenting Dysfunction in Chemically Dependent Women

William J Burns and Kayreen A Burns

The destructive impact of chemical abuse by a parent on other members of the family has been well documented in the literature[1,2]. Because the number of infants born to chemically abusing mothers is on the increase, there is a genuine concern about the quality of parenting by these mothers. It is reasonable to assume that the ignorance, naivety or irresponsibility that was involved in their use of drugs during pregnancy would carry over into their parenting. We know how important the mother's role is in the socio-emotional development of her infant. In the early dyadic interaction of mother and infant, when the early bases of development are laid, the mother's initiation of and response to her baby affect the likelihood of the occurance of specific infant behaviors. Newborn infants need to be carefully trained in how to interact socially. It is by first coacting with their mothers and fathers that they learn to initiate social interaction by themselves.

In a study of face-to-face communication, Kaye and Fogel[3] have shown that the mother's behavior affects the likelihood of the occurance of certain infant behaviors. After an initial phase of mother 'entraining' the rhythm of her infant's behavior, the infant behaviors gradually transfer to other contexts without maternal entrainment. Kaye interprets this as one of the dynamics for the origin of patterns of social behaviors.

In another study using normal dyads, Cohn and Tronick[4] found strong support for the hypothesis that mother–infant interaction is often initiated by the mother's positive elicitation of the infant. Secondly, Cohn and Tronick supported the notion that the mother's positive expression tends to precede the infant's positive expression. Finally, these authors showed that once the infant becomes positive, the mother tends to remain positive until the infant disengages.

In a similar vein, in a study of preterm infants, Marton, Minde and Ogilivie[5] found that mothers with more positive interpersonal histories have been shown to be more responsive to their infants' cues during interaction. Mothers of high-risk infants have been shown to endure greater stress than mothers of normal infants[6].

Mild psychopathology in the mother has been related to poor developmental progress. For instance, studies have shown a relationship between depression and adverse birth outcomes for an infant[7]. In the case of the major maternal psychopathology, the problem not only affects interaction and outcome but may be a cause of mental illness in the child. Massie's[8] description of the pathological interactions between psychotic mothers and their infants focuses on two lines of affective communication: the transmission of feeling by the mother to the child through facial expressions, and the baby's expression of emotional state. Massie's findings suggest that the psychotic mothers establish abnormal rules of interaction as a result of their own psychopathology. The infants adapt to these deviant demands and the adaptation becomes the source of deviant development. Thus, there are some maternal dimensions that are more convincing than others as causal factors in poor mother–infant interaction.

In a previous chapter[1] on the topic of mother–infant interactional pathology, we have reviewed the literature on the dysfunctional dynamics which lead to a pathological relationship. The potential for interactional difficulties is greater in the case of the drug-abusing mother than many other high-risk situations for social development, because the drug abuse affects both the mother and the infant. When both members of the dyad begin their relationship vulnerable to pathological interaction, not only is the risk for dysfunction higher, but also the prognosis for recovery is bleaker.

Add to these problems maternal ineptness, lack of personal resources including no spouse, and low socioeconomic status, and the risk of dysfunction is very high. In other words, there appears to be a complex of factors in a causal chain that leads to dysfunction. And an increase in the number of factors present leads to greater risk. In Figure 12.1 we present a model of what we consider to be the most significant of these risk factors in a flow chart of their hypothesized relationship to one another.

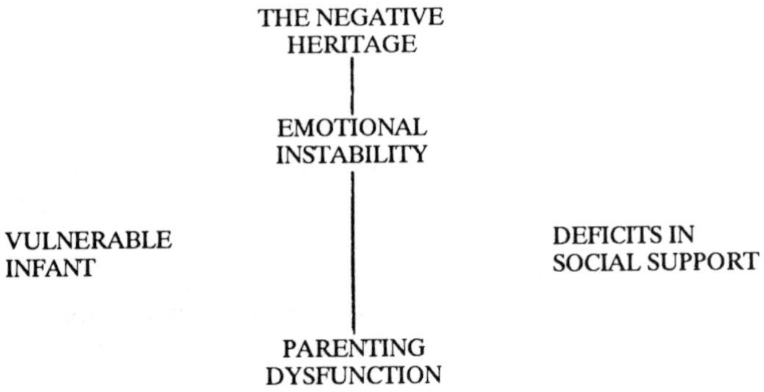

THE NEGATIVE
HERITAGE

EMOTIONAL
INSTABILITY

VULNERABLE
INFANT

DEFICITS IN
SOCIAL SUPPORT

PARENTING
DYSFUNCTION

Figure 12.1 Model of factors in parenting dysfunction

This model presents a direct link between the negative experience of being parented, the development of an unstable personality, and being a dysfunctional parent. The delivery of a vulnerable infant, and the absence of stable social support both complicate and intensify this dysfunctional parenting in the chemically abusing mother.

It is the purpose of this chapter to discuss some of these factors which seem to be precedents to dysfunctional parenting in drug-abusing mothers. We present hypothetical relationships between these factors in such a way that evidence may be gathered for and against these presumed linkages. Our four causal pathways are not new:

(1)   in a generational linkage from grandparents to parents negative methods of parenting are acquired;
(2)   the effect of the infant on the caregiver is intensified in the case of high-risk infancy;
(3)   absent or poor support from father, relatives or friends; and
(4)   personal, emotional instability in the mother.

THE GENERATIONAL LINKAGE

One of the long-range effects of being parented is to prepare an individual to become a parent. For better or for worse, parents transmit to their children a style of caretaking. As children grow up and make the transition from being a member of their parents' family to becoming parents themselves, they carry with them a heritage of child-rearing practices. The bulk of the literature on the intergenerational continuity of parenting has focused on the transmission of assets, positive values and productive support facilitated by lifelong affectional bonds[9]. The transmission of factors which may be precedents to dysfunctional parenting have also received some attention in matters such as child abuse. Berger[10] provides evidence for a multigenerational hypothesis of child abuse in which a complex of factors such as poverty, stress and personality interact with childhood history to increase or decrease the probability of child abuse in the next generation.

Taking another tack, some authors have shown that the offspring of parents with affective disorders develop deviations in personality such as lowered capacity for mutuality[11] which would put them at risk for dysfunctioning parenting. Connections have been made between parental use of alcohol and the adjustment of these children of alcoholics when they themselves become adults[12]. The complex array of precedents of dysfunctional parents which arise from the ways in which individuals themselves are parented are combined under the category *The Negative Heritage*.

MOTHER'S EMOTIONAL INSTABILITY

In the program at Northwestern we have come to expect a cluster of tendencies from mothers who use drugs. Mothers who give birth to infants while abusing drugs tend to be immature women who demonstrate an abnormal degree of egocentrism in the way they go about parenting. They frequently view the birth of the child as a gift for themselves and continue to interpret the child's growth and development in terms of their own needs. They have a great deal of difficulty understanding their infants' communications, since these communications are at first mostly expressions of the child's needs rather than responses to the mother's neediness. These mothers interpret their infant's attempts to communicate as demanding and inappropriate; and consequently they reject or criticize these early efforts to interact. At a time when their infant desperately needs encouragement to persist in social interaction, a message of discouragement is encountered instead. Parenting is experienced by the infant as a negative influence, as though the infants' growth and development were in competition with or at the expense of the mother's welfare.

Anecdotal accounts by these mothers relate their inability to make themselves get out of bed in the morning to care for their crying babies. Observation of their feeding practices show little sensitivity to the needs of the infant. Attempts to interact with toys often finds the play directed toward the mother's needs rather than that of her child. Researchers have not confirmed that these mothers are any different from their counterparts in a comparison group who use no drugs[19]. Whether they differ or not may be a moot issue, since they still need intervention and identifying them as drug-abusing mothers may be as good a way as any.

PERSONALITY

In the case of women who are chemical abusers, it is assumed that, in most instances, their use of drugs during pregnancy is not a temporary experimentation with drugs, but an enduring pathological dependence. If indeed their chemical abuse is a part of a consistent maladaptive life style, then their personality disorder places these mothers at high risk for associated problems such as mood and character disturbance. It is presumed that such character disturbances, although not as serious as psychosis, significantly affect the outcome of the infant.

For instance, at Northwestern we have evaluated the mother's emotional adjustment and found over 50% were moderately to severely depressed[13]. Any infant would feel the effect of having a depressed mother. Field[14] found that maternal depression was often reflected in depressive-like behaviors in infants.

In a small sample of mothers who were willing to complete the Minnesota Multiphasic Personality Inventory (MMPI) we found consistently highest scoring on Scale 4 (Figure 12.2, mean scale score = 69).

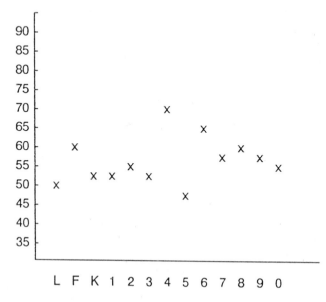

Figure 12.2 MMPI scores

Marks, Seeman and Haller[15] note that the criterion group on which Scale 4 was developed were people who had difficulty maintaining satisfactory personal relationships, profited little from experience in modifying their deficits and were poor at anticipating the consequences of their behavior. We found that of our sample of 10 cases, seven had T scores over 70. Five of these cases had greater than 70 T scores for Scale 4, three for Scale 8 and two for Scale 6. The criterion group for Scale 6 had paranoid symptoms and for Scale 8 thought disorders.

The 10 drug-abusing mothers who completed MMPI protocols, also filled out a Mother–Child Relationship Evaluation[16]. These were cocaine abusers between ages 20 and 37. The MMPI was completed during the third trimester of pregnancy and the MRCE in the first trimester after delivery. The MCRE is a 48-item self-rating of attitudes concerning parenting, e.g. 'If possible a mother should give her child all those things the mother never had'. Rating is on a 5-point scale from 'strongly agree' to 'strongly disagree.'

A priori factors result in scores for: maternal acceptance, overprotection, overindulgence, and rejection.

Acceptance

Mothers reported sincerity to affective expression, interest in the child's needs and development (somewhat a measure of attachment but also respect for individual personhood of child), e.g. children have rights of their own.

Overprotection (OP)

This is a failure in acceptance: an excessive control and prevention of the development of independent behavior, e.g. children cannot be trusted to do things for themselves.

Overindulgence (OI)

Excessive amount of time is given to the child while expressing a lack of parental control. Overdoing activities such as trips to zoo with excessive gratification of child, e.g. 'Somehow I cannot refuse any request my child makes', are included in this scale.

Rejection

This scale expresses denial of love and expression of hate by neglect, harshness, severity, brutality and strictness, e.g. when a child disobeys in school, the teacher should punish it.

Thus, **acceptance** is the only positive scale, **rejection** is the complete opposite of acceptance, and OP and OI reflect subtle forms of parental pathology which contain double messages of acceptance and rejection.

In the average profile of our 10 cases the principal elevation on this scale is the overprotection scale at the 87th percentile (although the overindulgence score is also slightly elevated at the 79th percentile). This is a good example of the profile on this scale we have found with each sample of chemically dependent mother records we have analyzed: acceptance and rejection scales in the average range and OP – OI elevated.

We interpret these elevations as an expression of these mothers' frustration in parenting. They seem to be saying that they vascillate between strictness and laxity which probably means vascillating between blaming or punishing and ignoring or neglecting. Such confused, inconsistent parenting would convey lack of attachment to the child. This lack of investment may be due to parental incompetence which is somewhat irreversible.

Mothers with MMPI scales over 70 tended to score lower on acceptance on the MCRE, while the 3 mothers with no scales over 70 all scored above the norm in acceptance on the MCRE. Likewise high overprotective scores tend to be those with more MMPI scales over 70. This association between maternal pathology and maternal attitude toward offspring we believe to be one of the links in the causal chain of factors leading to parenting pathology.

It is not a determining factor since some mothers with pathological scores report parenting attitudes in the normal range. But these 10 sample women show us some of the potential for deviant attitudes about parenting. This also would appear to reflect the Scale 8 mothers' failure to attach by being too strict and controlling.

Although such findings represent only data at a pilot level they point the way to some of the causal linkages in our model – principally the place of **maternal emotional development** and **maternal personality** as precedents of the mother–infant relationship and the development outcome of the infant.

SOCIAL SUPPORT DEFICITS

The critical role of mothering in the early social development of an infant becomes even more essential when that mother is a single parent. A majority (70–75% in our Northwestern group) of drug-abusing mothers are either unmarried or single mothers, who provide the bulk of parenting experience for their infant. Sixty-one percent of this Northwestern sample have never been married. Should that single parenting influence be dysfunctional, the impact is overwhelming for the infant.

Even in two parent families the father is often a drug abuser himself, or is a father who is not involved in parenting. Thus, the mother's personality and parenting skill is of significant importance for the social development of the infant. An inept mother who consistently chooses erroneous ways of relating and rearing may produce frustration in their infant. A mother who is lonely and isolated from family and other social support may turn toward the infant for human comfort a a time when the infant should be the one who can seek comfort from the mother.

When the family is intact (20% of our families have a married mother and father) and the mother's drug use is the only problem, an enormous burden may be shifted to the father. Only if he is a special person will he be able to fill such a void.

Normal family dynamics place considerable demands on the parents and children to cope with any special problems that arise[17]. When a new child is born, the father not only relates directly with the newborn infant, but also has indirect effects on the infant by affecting the mother's attitude toward herself and toward the infant[18]. It is considered to be a significant loss when the father is absent or psychologically unsupportive[19]. Thus, the scenario necessary for normal mother–infant interaction presumes the presence of a supportive father and husband. In the case of a drug-abusing mother, the situation calls for a heroic father, who can fill the roles of both mother and father when needed. The presence of such a supportive father could provide a positive coping force to stem the tide of dysfunction between mother and child. Sad to say, in the case of drug-abusing mothers, the heroic father is a rare breed. More often than not the fathers of these children are absent or drug abusers themselves.

Even in the case where the father is present, the relationship between mother and father may be unstable, or the birth of an infant with problems may lead to destabilization of an already tenuous relationship. A vicious downward cycle of family interaction may occur with crises. Such a process may end with total isolaton of the mother from all social resources, a situation which would be very risky for the infant when the mother–infant relationship deteriorates and allows for extremes of pathology, such as the cases of neonatal sexual abuse found in the NMH program[20].

It is not unusual for drug-abusing mothers to admit to child abuse, often in such a way that it seems they are oblivious to the serious nature of such abuse. Such was the case for several mothers in the Northwestern program who described their involvement in maternal–neonatal incest. All of these were mothers who were estranged from their sexual partners and who had demonstrated some role-confusion regarding sexual identity. These were lonely, socially isolated mothers, two of whom had been raped. The women were influenced to cease the incestuous activities with their infant sons when they became involved in psychotherapy. At the follow-up of these children at 3 and 4 years of age, they all show signs of significant emotional disturbance. Such destructive modes of parenting are often the combined result of heritage, emotional development and poor social support.

THE VULNERABLE INFANT

In addition to the direct effect of parenting on the infant, and the mutual effect of reciprocal exchange of behaviors in mother–infant interaction, we must consider the direct effect of the infant on its caregiver.

Especially through its ability to give progressively more discriminating attention and proximity-maintaining behavior an infant is able to draw the caregiver into a mutually productive relationship[21]. Likewise an infant who has experienced a high-risk delivery and who may be experiencing neonatal drug withdrawal as a neonate may have a negative effect on the mother, and therefore contribute indirectly to the mother's efforts at parenting. Researchers have demonstrated that a parents' perception that they have delivered an imperfect infant has a negative effect on their ability to take up the parenting role successfully[22]. Denial, sadness and sometimes shock are all combined with a need to cope with an unplanned imperfect child. Lack of adjustment can lead to thoughts and verbalization of rejection of the parenting role. Acts of rejection such as neglect and abandonment may occur at worst and, at best, the caretaking of the chemically abusing mothers may be half-hearted and lacking in genuine warmth.

For a number of years studies have documented the problems of other high-risk infants. For instance a number of studies have investigated the effect of high-risk infancy on mother–infant interaction. Field[23] and Goldberg[24] have documented the difficulties found in the mother–infant interaction where the infant is at risk. Not only does the birth of a high-risk infant confront a mother with a major stressor, but the infant may continue to show aberrant patterns of responsivity to mothering[25].

When a woman is told that the baby she is holding is 'high-risk', such a diagnosis alone may affect the way the woman relates to the baby, even if it is not true the baby is high-risk[26].

Bakeman and Brown[27] found that high-risk infants do not take as much responsibility for maintaining the mother–infant dialogue as do normal infants. Therefore, maintaining the flow of communication falls disproportionately on the mother. It has also been found that high-risk infants smile a proportionately less amount of time during mother–infant interaction than normal infants[6]. Willie[28] found that an infants' perinatal medical status has an impact on attachment patterns and length of cry which in turn influences the mother–infant relationship.

In studies which have collected information on mother–infant interactions of high-risk infants at several age levels, mixed findings have been obtained. Field, Dempsey and Shuman[29] did ratings of face-to-face interactions of three groups of infants: healthy term, preterm with respiratory distress and post-term. When the infants were 4 months of age, they found significant interactional difficulties. At one year of age, these authors found no group differences using the Ainsworth procedures. However, at 2 years of age, differences were again evident in infant – mother interaction.

Als[30] pointed out that each mother – infant dyad has a given configuration of personal, social, cultural and biological variables which lead to a unique experience of communication and mutual regulation. The earlier that an examiner identifies the interactive goals of a particular dyad, the better that examiner may develop intervention strategies which may diminish the deviance in social interaction often found in dyads with a high-risk infant. The birth of an infant with defects may sap maternal and infant energies that should be devoted to social interaction. In turn the lack of success in mother – infant interaction may negatively affect developmental outcome of the infant.

There develops a downward spiral of developmental and social dysfunction where there should have been mutual enhancement. The successful negotiation of affective reciprocity is an essential aspect of realizing the full potential of an infant with birth defects. The infant's medical condition may produce a drain on the developmental process and the interactive system with the mother. Als[30] has shown that assessing the quality of each interaction in the mother – infant system is the prerequisite to accurate intervention. The common thread in all these findings is that high-risk infancy is involved in the causal chain that produces difficulties in the mother – infant interaction.

Our studies and those of others have shown that infants of chemically dependent mothers have neurobehavioral problems during the newborn period. The mother – infant interactions of these dyads also indicate difficulties. One would expect that deficits in developmental progress would follow. The outcome literature, however, does not support this expectation. Many researchers report normal developmental progress beyond the newborn period[31 – 34].

There are, however, two studies in the literature that reported significantly poorer developmental outcome for drug-exposed children[35,36]. Both of these studies had over 40 subjects in their drug-exposed groups. Because data collection in this population is fraught with so many complications, large subject pools are necessary in order to capture the flavor of the 'typical' child who experienced prenatal drug exposure. It is our experience that the children whom we have complete longitudinal data on are the children of our most stable mothers or the mothers who are inadequate, but have attached themselves to us for continued support and child-rearing advice.

Neither of these groups are 'typical' of the drug-abusing population, yet they comprise the majority of our longitudinal data pool.

CONCLUSIONS

We propose that each of these four factors in our causal pathway have an influence on the presence and intensity of the dysfunction in parenting. As the flow chart in Figure 12.1 indicates the factors of 'negative heritage' and 'emotional instability' have a proposed direct and mutually cumulative effect. For example, a mother who has been abused by her own parent, is more likely to experience personal instability in her own emotional development and to become a dysfunctional parent as a direct result of the social trauma and personal maladjustment. The more current factors of 'social support deficits' and 'vulnerable infant' indirectly affect parenting through 'emotional stability' or more directly. For example, a mother whose husband does not participate in parenting may feel isolated and needy to the extent that she sexually abuses her infant as a way of filling the void in her social life. Thus, dysfunctional parenting is an indirect result of lack of social support. More directly, the infant might use irritability to try to obtain the mother's attention, and directly trigger rejection.

It is our hypothesis that the more direct effects are more potent in producing dysfunctional parenting. It also seem reasonable to hypothesize that the more factors involved the greater the cumulative risk of dysfunction. For instance, when a mother has experienced a negative heritage, it only makes it more difficult for her to extend herself to a vulnerable child.

And finally the intensity of the dysfunction is assumed to be related to the intensity of the precedents. This model is being tested in our project at Northwestern. We offer it as a testable model for others. In the interim before evidence is available, we hope that it will serve to spark research. Some programs have offered clinical services based on the above hypotheses[37]. Preventative efforts with these mothers and their infants have focused on a combination of physical, emotional and social development of the children and the mothers' role in fostering their development.

REFERENCES

1. Burns, W. (1986). Psychopathology of mother–infant interaction. In Chasnoff, I. (ed.) *Drug Use in Pregnancy: Mother and Child*, pp. 106–116. (Lancaster: MTP Press Ltd)
2. West, M. and Prinz, R. (1987). Parental alcoholism and childhood psychopathology. *Psychol. Bull.*, **102**, 204–18
3. Kaye, K. and Fogel, A. (1980). The temporal structure of face-to-face communication between mothers and infants. *Devel. Psychol.*, **16**, 454–64
4. Cohn, J. and Tronick, E. (1987). Mother–infant face to face interaction: the sequence of dyadic states at 3, 6 and 9 months. *Devel. Psychol.*, **23**, 68–77

5. Marton, P., Minde, K. and Ogilvie, J. (1981). Mother–infant interactions in the premature nursery: a sequential analysis. In Friedman, S. and Sigman, M.N. (eds.) *Preterm Birth and Psychological Development*, pp. 179–205. (New York: Academic Press)
6. Laney, M. and Sandler, H. (1982). Relationships among maternal stress, infant status and mother–infant interactions. In Lipsitt, L.P. and Fields, T.M. (eds.). *Infant Behavior and Development: Perinatal Risk and Newborn Behavior*, pp. 139–52. (Norwood NJ: Ablex Publishing Corp)
7. Zuckerman, B.H. and Beardslee, W. (1987). Maternal depression: a concern for pediatricians. *Pediatrics*, **79**, 110–17
8. Massie, H. (1982). Affective development and the organization of mother–infant behavior from the perspective of psychopathology. In Tronick, E.Z. (ed.). *Social Interchange in Infancy*, pp. 161–82. (Baltimore: University Park Press)
9. Moss, N., Abrahamowitz, S.I. and Rascusin, G. (1985). Parental heritage: progress and prospect. In L'Abate, L. (ed.) *The Handbook of Family Psychology and Therapy*, pp. 499–522. (Homewood, Illinois: The Dorsey Press)
10. Berger, A. (1985). Characteristics of abusing families. In L'Abate, L. (ed.) *The Handbook of Family Psychology and Therapy*, pp. 900–36. (Homewood, Illinois: The Dorsey Press)
11. Beardslee, W., Schultz, L. and Selman, R. (1987). Level of social–cognitive development, adaptive functioning, and DSM-III diagnoses in adolescent offspring of parents with affective disorders: implications of the development of the capacity for mutuality. *Devel. Psychol.*, **23**, 807–15
12. Black, C. (1981). *It Will Never Happen To Me: Children of Alcoholics as Youngsters, Adolescents, and Adults*. (Rutherford, N.J.: Thomas, W., Perrin, Inc.)
13. Burns, K., Melamed, J., Burns, W., Chasnoff, I. and Hatcher, R. (1985). Chemical dependency and depression in pregnancy. *J. Clin. Psychol.*, **41**. 851–54
14. Field, T. (1984). Perinatal risk factors for infant depression. In Call, J., Galenson, E. and Tyson, R. (eds.) *Frontiers of Infant Psychiatry*, Vol. II, pp. 152–59. (New York: Basic Books, Inc.)
15. Marks, P., Seeman, W. and Haller, D. (1974). *The Actuarial Use of the MMPI with Adolescents and Adults*. (Baltimore: Williams & Wilkins)
16. Roth, R. (1961). *The Mother–Child Relationship Evaluation*. (Los Angeles: Western Psychol. Services)
17. Dunn, J. and Mann, P. (1985). Becoming a family member: family conflict and the development of social understanding in the second year. *Child Devel.*, **56**, 480–92
18. Parke, R.D. (1979). Perspectives on father–infant interaction. In Osofsky, J. (ed.) *Handbook of Infant Development*, pp. 549–90. (New York: John Wiley)
19. Jeremy, R.J. and Bernstein, V.J. (1984). Dyads at risk: methadone-maintained women and their four-month-old infants. *Child Devel.*, **55**, 1141–54
20. Chasnoff, I., Burns, W., Schnoll, S., Burns, W., Chisum, G. and Kyle-Spore, L. (1986). Maternal-neonatal incest. *Am. J. Orthopsychiatr.*, **56**, 577–80
21. Bell, R.Q. (1974). Contributions of human infants to caregiving and social interaction. In Lewis, M. and Rosenblum, L. (eds.) *The Effect of the Infant on its Caregiver*, pp. 1–20. (New York: John Wiley)
22. Tymchuk, A.J. (1979). *Parent and Family Therapy*. (New York: SP Medical & Scientific Books)
23. Field, T.M. (1979). Interaction patterns of preterm and term infants. In Field, T.M., Sostek, A.M., Goldberg, S. and Shuman, H. (eds.) *Infants Born at Risk*, pp. 333–56. (New York: SP Medical and Scientific Books)
24. Goldberg, S. (1978). Prematurity-effects on parent–infant interaction. *J. Pediatr. Psychol.*, **3**, 137–44
25. Lewis, M., Thompson, R., Meisels, S., Plunkett, J., Steifel, G., Pasick, P. and Roloff, D. (1984). Developmental vulnerability of infants born at severe risk. Paper presented at the *Fourth International Conference on Infant Studies*. New York, April, 1984
26. Stern, M. and Hildebrandt, K. (1986). Prematurity stereotyping: Effects on mother–infant interaction. *Child Devel.*, **57**, 309–15

27. Bakeman, R. and Brown, J.V. (1980). Analyzing behavioral sequences: differences between preterm and full-term infant–mother dyads during the first months of life. In Savin, D. *et al.* (eds.) *The Exceptional Infant*, Vol. 4, pp. 271–99. (Bruner/Mazel: New York)
28. Willie, D. (1987). Prematurity, mother–infant interaction and attachment. Paper presented at the *Biennial Meeting of the Society for Research in Child Development*, Baltimore, MD., April 1987
29. Field, T., Dempsey, J. and Shuman, H. (1981). Developmental follow-up of pre- and post-term infants. In Friedman, S. and Sigman, M. (eds.) *Preterm Birth and Psychological Development*, pp. 299–312. (New York: Academic Press)
30. Als, H. (1982). The unfolding of behavioral organization in the face of a biological violation. In Tronick, E.Z. (ed.) *Social Interchange in Infancy*, pp. 125–60. (Baltimore: University Park Press)
31. Kallenbach, K. and Finnegan, L. (1986). Neonatal abstinence syndrome, pharmacotherapy and developmental outcome. *Neurobehav. Toxicol. Teratol.*, **8**, 353–5
32. Suffet, F. and Brotman, R. (1984). A comprehensive care program for pregnant addicts: obstetrical, neonatal and child development outcomes. *Int. J. Addict.*, **19**, 199–219
33. Fried, P. (1982). Marijuana use be pregnant women and effects on offspring: An update. *Neurobehav. Toxicol. Teratol.*, **4**, 451–4
34. Lifschultz, M., Wilson, G., Smith, E. and Desmond, M. (1985). Factors affecting head growth and intellectual function in children of drug addicts. *Pediatrics*, **75**, 269–74
35. Billing, L., Eriksson, M., Steneroth, G. and Zetterstrom, R. (1985). Pre-school children of amphetamine-addicted mothers. In Somatic and psychomotor development. *Acta. Paediatr. Scand.*, **74**, 179–84
36. Rosen, T. and Johnson, H. (1982). Children of methadone-maintained mothers: Follow-up to 18 months of age. *J. Pediatr.*, **101**, 192–6
37. Lief, N. (1985). The drug user as a parent: Intervening with special populations. *Int. J. Addict.*, **20**, 63–97

13

Viral Hepatitis in Pregnancy

Dietra Delaplane Millard

Pregnant women who have acute or chronic viral hepatitis during pregnancy can transmit the infecting virus to their offspring. Although many of these women will have mild or asymptomatic disease, the infant may become infected depending on the virus involved. In the case of hepatitis B, many of these infants will develop chronic liver disease or even hepatoma, as well as have the potential to transmit the disease within the household if they do not receive proper prophylaxis in the neonatal period. It is essential for those of us who care for pregnant women and neonates to have a working understanding of viral hepatitis to appropriately treat these patients to inhibit the spread of this disease.

Acute viral hepatitis occurs infrequently in pregnant women in the USA, although the precise frequency is unknown since many cases are subclinical and escape detection. In an urban hospital in Chicago serving nearly equal numbers of indigent and private obstetrical patients, only six cases of acute viral hepatitis were identified in pregnant women over the last three years, during which time there were 12,748 deliveries. This suggests an incidence of approximately 1:2000 births in this population. Chronic hepatitis occurs more frequently in parturient women in the Chicago population, with 21 cases recognized in the last three years. This is most commonly due to chronic asymptomatic carriage of hepatitis B (18 cases), with two additional cases of chronic active hepatitis B and one case of chronic non-A, non-B hepatitis. But these numbers represent minimum estimates since only women at risk for hepatitis B are screened at this institution. Undoubtedly, the incidence is actually higher, especially in impoverished populations with poor hygenic conditions.

Most women with either acute or chronic viral hepatitis have successful pregnancies and deliver at term although those from underdeveloped countries or those with nutritional deficiecies may have a higher morbidity[1-5]. This chapter will review the known causes of viral hepatitis, the effect of such infections on the pregnant woman and her offspring, screening criteria for pregnant women at risk for hepatitis, and current recommendations for prophylactic treatment of the newborn.

ETIOLOGY

At present there are three common types of viral hepatitis: hepatitis A, hepatitis B, and non-A, non-B hepatitis. A fourth type of hepatitis is now recognized called hepatitis D (delta agent)[6]. The latter disease is only seen in some patients with hepatitis B infection as the delta agent requires hepatitis B virus for replication. Since infection with the delta agent has epidemiologic characteristics and clinical effects similar to hepatitis B[7-8], it will be included in the discussion of hepatitis B.

Specific characteristics of each of the three common types of viral hepatitis are shown in Table 13.1.

Table 13.1 Characteristics of common types of viral hepatitis

Characteristics	Hepatitis A	Hepatitis B	Non-A, non-B
Virus type	RNA	DNA	Unknown
Incubation period	2–8 weeks	1–6 months	1–6 months
Vertical transmission to fetus	Rare, if ever	Common	Probable
Maximum infectivity	Prodrome	HBsAg + and HBeAg*	Prodrome
Carrier state	No	5–10%	10–50%
Chronic disease	No	CPH* and CAH**	CPH* and CAH**
		Cirrhosis and/or hepatoma late complications	

*   Chronic persistent hepatitis
** Chronic active hepatitis

Hepatitis A

Hepatitis A virus (HAV) is transmitted primarily via the fecal–oral route, and typicaly causes a 'flu-like' illness or asymptomatic infection. The patient is most contagious early in the course of the infection before symptoms are appreciated. Although viremia occurs briefly just prior to onset of symptoms, acute infection with HAV in a pregnant woman does not pose a threat to a fetus[9]. Neither a chronic form of HAV nor a carrier state of HAV is recognized.

Hepatitis B

Hepatitis B virus (HBV) is transmissible by multiple routes including fecal–oral and parenteral exposure to blood or body fluids infected with HBV. Acute HBV infection is clinically similar to HAV infection but may be more serious because of chronic sequelae of HBV. About 5–10% of adults with acute HBV recover from symptoms of the disease but continue to carry HBV (chronic carrier state). Many of these will develop chronic persistent or chronic active hepatitis, which often progresses to hepatoma[10]. HBV can be transmitted from both acutely and chronically infected persons to their contacts. Vertical transmission of HBV from infected mother to newborn occurs in 15–70% of cases, depending on geographic location and socio-economic and serologic status of the mother[9,11–14]. Although several factors contribute to the variable transmission rates observed, it appears from several studies that women with serum positive for HBe antigen more frequently transmit the infection to the infant[15,16].

In infants who acquire HBV vertically at birth, approximately 85 percent become carriers of HBV with a high risk of developing cirrhosis and hepatoma[16]. Since prompt immunoprophylaxis of infants born to HBV-infected women has been shown to be extremely effective[17], it is essential for physicians and caretakers of pregnant women to be familiar with risk factors for HBV and to identify infected women prenatally so that their offspring receive appropriate care in the immediate perinatal period.

Non-A, non-B Hepatitis

Non-A, non-B hepatitis is caused by at least two distinct agents[18] and, likely, by multiple agents[19]. It is the most frequent cause of post-transfusion hepatitis[20,21] but may be transmitted by both parenteral and fecal–oral[22–24] routes. Acute non-A, non-B hepatitis frequently causes mild, anicteric disease, but, like HBV infections, there is both a carrier state and/or chronic form of non-A, non-B infection, and cirrhosis and progressive hepatic failure are recognized complications of this infection in adults[25]. Transmission of non-A, non-B hepatitis vertically from mother to infant probably occurs[9,26] but the extent of long-term sequelae of this infection in infants will remain unknown until a reliable serologic marker is developed.

SEROLOGIC MARKERS

Serologic markers are readily available to diagnose both hepatitis A and hepatitis B infections (Table 13.2), but there are no serologic tests available for non-A, non-B hepatitis.

Table 13.2 Serologic markers of viral hepatitis

Marker	Abbreviation
Hepatitis A virus	HAV
Hepatitis A antibody	anti-HAV
Hepatitis B virus	HBV
Hepatitis B surface antigen	HBsAg
Hepatitis B surface antibody	anti-HBs
Hepatitis B core antibody	anti-HBc
Hepatitis B e antigen	HBeAg
Hepatitis B e antibody	anti-HBe

Hepatitis A

The chronology of hepatitis A infection is shown in Figure 13.1. Antibody to hepatitis A (anti-HAV) becomes detectable in serum at about the same time that symptoms become apparent. In the early stages of the disease, the antibody is of the IgM type (anti-HAV-IgM), but IgG predominates in the months following and probably persists for life, providing protection against reinfection. Detection of anti-HAV-IgM is diagnostic of acute hepatitis A infection.

Hepatitis B

There are multiple serologic markers for hepatitis B (Table 13.3) and each of these is present at different times in the course of this infection. Figure 13.2 depicts the chronology of acute hepatitis B infection with recovery, Figure 13.3 shows the chronology of such an infection followed by chronic asymptomatic carriage of HBV, and Figure 13.4 shows acute HBV with progression to chronic active hepatitis.

Detailed discussions of the components of the hepatitis B virus[27] and its serologic markers[28] have been published elsewhere and will be reviewed here briefly.

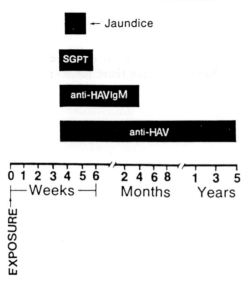

Figure 13.1 Chronology of symptoms, elevated liver function tests, and serologic markers in acute hepatitis A

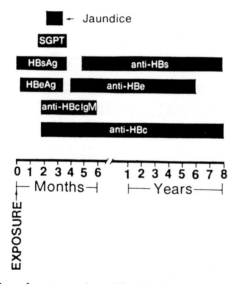

Figure 13.2 Chronology of symptoms, elevated liver function tests, and serologic markers in acute hepatitis B with recovery

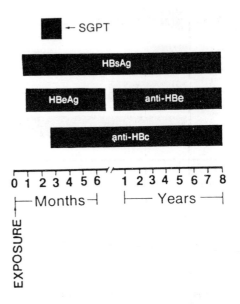

Figure 13.3 Chronology of elevated liver function tests and serologic markers in chronic carriage of hepatitis B

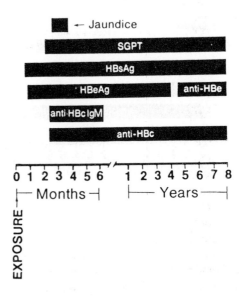

Figure 13.4 Chronology of elevated liver function tests and serologic markers in chronic active hepatitis B

Table 13.3 Interpretation of serologic markers of hepatitis B infection and need for prophylaxis of infant

Maternal serologic markers			Immunoprophylaxis of infant
HBsAg	anti-HBs	anti-HBc	
1. +	−	−	yes
2. +	−	+	yes
3. +	+	+	yes
4. −	−	+	no*
5. −	+	+	no
6. −	+	−	no

* yes if anti-HBc is of IgM type

Interpretation

1. Early acute infection or chronic carrier state
2. Early acute infection if anti-HBc is of IgM type: chronic infection if anti-HBc is of IgG type
3. Late acute infection with crossover of HBsAg and anti-HBs, or chronic carrier state with heterotypic antibody (rare)
4. 'Core window' in acute infection if anti-HBc is of IgM type: recovery from acute infection in past if anti-HBc is of IgG type (anti-HBs has waned)
5. Recovery from acute infection in past
6. Immunity from acute infection in past (anti-HBc has waned) or person has received passive immunity from hepatitis B immunoglobulin or has active immunity from hepatitis B vaccine

Hepatitis B surface antigen (HBsAg) is a protein fragment of the HBv and usually is detectable in serum after an incubation period of 1–6 months. HBsAg typically peaks at the onset of symptoms then disappears 1–2 months later. Hepatitis B surface antibody (anti-HBs) appears the following month and indicates recovery and immunity to HBV. Current technology does not permit serologic measurement of the hepatitis B core antigen, but the hepatitis B core antibody (anti-HBc) is detectable early in the course of the infection and frequently persists in chronic forms of the disease and in patients who have recovered. In most cases of acute HBV there is a gap in time, usually 2–4 weeks, between the disappearance of HBsAg and the appearance of anti-HBs. During this time, commonly called the 'core window', neither HBsAg nor anti-HBs is detectable but antibody to the core antigen (anti-HBc) is present. Present laboratory methods can determine that this is of the IgM type (anti-HBc-IgM) and confirm the diagnosis of acute HBV infection. If anti-HBc is present but anti-HBc-IgM is not detectable, it is likely the person has recovered from the acute hepatitis B

179

infection in the past (anti-HBs is also present) or that the person has a chronic form of HBV infection (HBsAg is also present).

Although its origin remains unclear, hepatitis B e antigen (HBeAg) is detectable in the serum of some patients with acute infection or chronic carriage of HBV, coincident with the presence of HBsAg. Its significance is predominantly epidemiologic indicating that large quantities of virus are present with a high degree of infectivity for contacts[15,29,30]. The antibody to HBe antigen (anti-HBe) appears at about the same time as anti-HBs. But all persons with HBsAg, whether HBeAg is present or not, should be considered contagious. Therefore, measurement of maternal HBeAg or anti-HBe is not necessary for clinical management of the newborn to the HBsAg-positive mother.

Interpreting of serologic markers for hepatitis B can be difficult and confusing. Table 13.3 summarizes a variety of combinations of serologic results with an interpretation of each. Serologic tests taken early in the pregnancy that indicate an acute infection should be repeated shortly before delivery to assure proper care of the infant. Since hepatitis D virus requires HBV for replication, serologies for HBV are monitored.

Non-A, Non-B Hepatitis

The diagnosis of non-A, non-B hepatitis necessitates eliminating hepatitis A or hepatitis B as a cause as well as other viral agents that cause hepatitis, specifically cytomegalovirus or Epstein–Barr virus. There are no specific serologic markers for non-A, non-B infection and elevation of liver enzymes may wax and wane[19].

PREGNANCY AND PERINATAL TRANSMISSION OF VIRAL HEPATITIS

Hepatitis A

Hepatitis A infection commonly occurs in childhood and adolescence and is more prevalent in developing countries where living conditions are crowded, hygiene is poor, and contaminated food or water facilitate spread of the disease. Although pregnant women from impoverished countries who contract hepatitis A infection may have an increased mortality and morbidity from this disease[2-4], reports from industrialized countries suggest that the course and outcome of maternal disease is not affected by the pregnancy[9,31,32]. One study suggests an increased incidence of prematurity when

HAV infection is contracted late in pregnancy, but found no evidence that hepatitis A during pregnancy causes birth defects[31].

Hepatitis A is rarely, if ever, transmitted from a pregnant mother to her baby, whether the mother's infection occurs early or late in pregnancy[9].

Serologic evaluation of babies born to these women sometimes shows passive anti-HAV when the mother's disease occurred early in pregnancy, but no clinical or laboratory evidence of hepatitis is found in most cases.

Hepatitis B

In contrast to acute HAV infections in pregnant women, transmission of HBV from mother to infant is common[9,11,12,16]. Women who are chronic carriers of HBV and those with acute HBV in the month before or after delivery are more likely to transmit the HBV to their offspring than those who have acute HBV infection in the first or second trimester and then recover[33,34]. Thus, any woman who is HBsAg-positive at the time of delivery has a high chance of infecting her infant. Although mothers who have both HBsAg and HBeAg pose the greatest threat to their offspring (approximately 85% will become infected and about 85% of these infants will become chronic carriers)[16], severe, even fatal infections have been reported in infants whose mothers were chronic HBsAg carriers without HBeAg[35]. Proper immunoprophylaxis of the newborn infant is essential to all babies born to mothers with HBsAg, regardless of HBeAg results[36].

The vast majority of infants born to mothers with acute or chronic HBV appear healthy and are not jaundiced at birth. Most of those who acquire HBV from their mothers are exposed in the intrapartum period[12,37]. Serial serologic studies of such babies have demonstrated that most infants become HBsAg positive between 2–4 months of age[38,39], corresponding to the known incubation period for HBV. Occasional infants develop anti-HBs at about the same time, suggesting peripartum exposure to HBV with subsequent immunity.

Only rarely does an infant born to a mother with HBV show evidence of HBV infection at birth[37], suggesting intrauterine acquisition of the virus. The presence of HBsAg in cord blood shows no correlation with the subsequent appearance of antigenemia in the infant[12]. As well, the majority of newborns with HBsAg-positive cord blood have no detectable antigen in blood obtained from a peripheral vein. Thus, the occasional detection of HBsAg in cord blood may reflect contamination with maternal blood during collection or leakage of blood across the placenta from mother to infant[40] during labor but not active intrauterine acquisition of HBV.

The route of transmission of HBV from mother to infant remains unclear, but high concentrations of HBsAg are detected in blood of both acutely and chronically infected persons and in lower levels in almost all body fluids[41]. This includes amniotic fluid and vaginal fluid of pregnant women, cord blood and gastric contents of the newborn, and breast milk of the infected woman post-partum[12]. Thus transmission could occur by multiple routes including the infant swallowing amniotic fluid and/or maternal blood, leakage of maternal blood across the placenta into the infant *in utero* or during labor, invasion through mucous membranes or minor abrasions during delivery, or post-partum through breastfeeding or during close contact with mother and other family members likely to be infected.

There is no evidence that Caesarean delivery protects the infant from HBV infection. In a study from Hong Kong, infants delivered by Caesarean section became infected as readily as those delivered vaginally[12]. In an animal study of HBV infection in a pregnant chimpanzee, the baby chimpanzee became infected despite Caesarean delivery and complete isolation from the mother[42]. These circumstances were also described in the first case report of vertical transmission of hepatitis by Stokes *et al.* more than three decades ago[43]. Because of the high prevalence of HBsAg positivity in vaginal fluid and gastric aspirates of the infant at birth, some investigators suggest the oral route during delivery as the most likely means of mother-to-infant transmission of HBV[12]. It is likely that more than one route plays a role in transmission of this infection from mother to baby.

Although minimal data are published regarding the transmissibility of the delta agent, Italian investigators have reported perinatal transmission of hepatitis B and hepatitis D from mother to infant[44]. It is unclear what contribution the delta agent has in the course of HBV infections in newborns.

Non-A, Non-B Hepatitis

Very little is also known about the transmission of non-A, non-B hepatitis from mother to infant. The lack of specific serologic markers for this infection have made it difficult to study the route and rate of maternal–infant transmission. A prospective study of 12 women with non-A, non-B hepatitis during pregnancy and their offspring showed transiently elevated liver enzymes in six of the infants[9], suggesting that the agent(s) causing non-A, non-B hepatitis is transmissible from the gravid woman to her infant. From this study, it also appears that acute non-A, non-B hepatitis in the third trimester is associated with a higher rate of transmission than when it occurs earlier[9]. There are no published data regarding transmission rate of this disease from mothers with chronic non-A, non-B disease to their infants.

One infant born at our institution to a mother with chronic non-A, non-B hepatitis preceding the pregnancy was healthy at delivery and had no documented elevation of serum glutamic pyruvic transaminase (SGPT) in the first 12 months of life. (The infant was given empiric immunoprophylaxis with standard immune globulin in the delivery room.) The long-term consequences of acute non-A, non-B hepatitis in infants are unknown at present.

SCREENING CRITERIA FOR PREGNANT WOMEN

Because immunoprophylaxis of the neonate is efficacious in preventing the maternal–fetal transmission of hepatitis B[17,45–47], it is imperative that women with acute or chronic viral hepatitis be identified during pregnancy. This permits the obstetrician to notify the pediatricians before the infant is born. The more promptly the infant receives immunoprophylaxis the less likely (s)he is to acquire hepatitis[48].

Table 13.4 Prevalence of hepatitis B virus infection in various population groups*

Population group	Prevalence of serologic markers of HBV infection	
	HBsAg* (%)	All markers (%)
Immigrants from areas of HBV endemicity	13	70–85
Residents at institutions for the mentally retarded	10–20	35–80
Intravenous drug abusers	7	60–80
Homosexual males	6	35–80
Household contacts of HBv carriers	3–6	30–60
Hemodialysis patients	3–10	20–80
Health care workers with frequent blood contact	1–2	15–30
Healthy adults	0.3	3–5

* Adapted from MMWR, **31**, 318 (1982)

The prevalence of HBsAg in healthy adults in the United States is approximately 0.3%[49]. The prevalence of serologic markers for HBV infection in specific populations in the USA is shown in Table 13.4. At least those groups with HBsAg prevalence exceeding one percent are at high risk for HBV infection and should be screened prenatally[50] (Table 13.5). Because routine screening of all pregnant women for HBV infection has been shown to be cost-effective[51], it is anticipated that this will be adopted as standard prenatal care in the near future.

Proper screening for hepatitis B includes testing for HBsAg and anti-HBc-IgM. Interpretation of the results of this serologic screen is reviewed in Table 13.3.

Table 13.5 Women at risk for chronic HBsAg carriage for whom prenatal screening for HBV is recommended

1. Those with a current or previous history of clinical hepatitis
2. Immigrant women from areas of high HBV endemicity, particularly Asia, Africa, Alaska (Eskimos), and Pacific Islands
3. Those who have received or work with blood products
4. Those whose husbands are hemophiliacs
5. Those who have been rejected as blood donors
6. Those who are associated with hemodialysis units or institutions for the retarded as patients or staff
7. Health and dental care personnel with exposure to blood
8. Those who are known parenteral drug abusers and/or prostitutes
9. Those with multiple episodes of sexually transmitted diseases
10. Those with a household member or sexual partner with hepatitis B

* Adapted from MMWR, **43**, 314 (1985)

IMMUNOPROPHYLAXIS AND CARE OF THE NEONATE

Hepatitis A

Although transmission of HAV from mother to infant has not been documented, some hepatologists suggest immunoprophylaxis of the neonate with a single dose of standard immune serum globulin (ISG), 0.5 ml intramuscularly (i.m.) if the mother has acute HAV at the time of delivery[9]. The efficacy of this has not been established and the risk of transmission without prophylaxis appears quite low.

Enteric precautions are mandatory for all persons with acute HAV, but separation of the mother and infant is unnecessary[52]. Because HAV is spread by the fecal–oral route, the mother should be instructed explicitly about the need for careful handwashing. There is no apparent risk to breast feeding.

Hepatitis B

Infants born to mothers with acute or chronic HBV infections are usually healthy at birth with appropriate growth parameters[9,34]. Typically, there is no clinical, laboratory, or serologic evidence of infection in the neonatal period. However, combined treatment with both hepatitis B immune globulin (HBIG) and hepatitis B vaccine (HBvac) provides maximum immuno-prophylaxis for the infant[17,45-47]. In the delivery room immediately after birth, the infant is frequently contaminated with maternal blood and vaginal secretions containing HBV[12]. All medical personnel caring for the mother and/or infant in the delivery suite should adhere to proper infection control measures for contaminated blood and body fluids. It is our practice to aspirate the infant's gastric contents and discard properly, and then bathe the infant promptly. We then draw a hepatitis B screen (HBsAg, anti-HBs, anti-HBc) from a peripheral vein of the infant and inject HBIG i.m. before the infant leaves the delivery suite. The recommended dose of HBIG is 0.5 ml[50].

To be most efficacious, all three doses of the HBvac are important to provide immunity to HBV infection[53,54]. The first dose of HBvac should be administered prior to hospital discharge after obtaining results of the infant's HBV screen. In most cases, all three serologic tests are negative. If HBsAg is already present, HBvac (an expensive agent) is not warranted. Trials in adults who are HBsAg positive showed HBvac to be safe but not effective in eliminating HBsAg[55]. Others suggest that serologic screening of the infant who is HBsAg positive should not preclude HBvac administration, and that the vaccine may be helpful in recovery from a presumed intrauterine HBV infection[56].

It is imperative that these infants receive close follow-up to ensure completion of the vaccine series. (The second and third doses of HBvac should be given at 1 month and 6 months of age.) As well, we suggest HBV screening for all household contacts of the mother, specifically any other offspring[15], and vaccination for any who do not yet have serologic evidence of infection. It is suggested that all vaccinated infants have repeated serologic testing at 9-12 months of age to verify the efficacy of the immuno-prophylaxis. The duration of immunity is unknown and there are no current recommendations regarding need for booster shots of HBvac for infants or adults.

We administer HBIG in the delivery room regardless of the infant's gestational age, but initiate the vaccine at 32 weeks post-conceptional age if the baby is younger than that at birth. HBvac may be administered concurrently with HBIG or other vaccines but injections should be at different sites[50].

It is not necessary to isolate infants born to HBsAg positive mothers once they are bathed and have received their HBIG, although blood and body fluid precautions should be exercised rigorously in caring for the mother prenatally and in the post-partum period[52]. We encourage the mother and her offspring to room-in together.

Whether breastfeeding is risky to the infant whose mother is HBsAg positive is unknown. Although HBsAg can be detected in breast milk[12] posing an ongoing exposure to HBV for the infant, studies from an endemic region have not confirmed an increased risk of HBV in breastfed infants[57]. It is important to consider both the potential benefits of breastfeeding and the possible risks of ongoing HBV exposure when discussing this issue with a mother. It is our practice to advise a mother against breastfeeding because of concern that additional viral exposure may lead to unsuccessful prophylaxis and life-long chronic hepatic disease in the infant. Others, including Dr Saul Krugman, do not discourage breastfeeding, particularly in developing countries where the benefits are so important[58].

Non-A, Non-B Hepatitis

Because some infants born to mothers with non-A, non-B hepatitis have had elevation of hepatic enzyme activity in the first few months[9], it is suggested that the infant receive ISG promptly after birth. This should be given again at 2 and 4 months of age because of the long incubation period for non-A, non-B hepatitis and presumed intrapartum transmission. Measurement of the infant's SGPT at 3 and 5 months is reasonable to determine if the infant has non-A, non-B infection. Enteric spread of this disease has been reported[22-24], so it is important to maintain appropriate infection control measures, but separation of mother and infant is not needed. The risk of breastfeeding is unknown.

REFERENCES

1. Borhanmanesh, F., Haghighi, P., Hekmat, K., Rezaizadeh, K. and Ghavami, A.G. (1973). Viral hepatitis during pregnancy: severity and effect on gestation. *Gastroenterology*, **64**, 304–12
2. Christie, A.B., Allam, A.A., Aref, M.K., El Muntasser, I.H. and El-Nageh, M. (1976). Pregnancy hepatitis in Libya. *Lancet*, **2**, 827–9
3. Shwer, M. and Moosa, A. (1979). The effects of hepatitis A and B in pregnancy on mother and fetus. *S. Afr. Med. J.*, **54**, 10925
4. Akhtar, K.A.K. and Akhtar, M.A. (1979). Viral hepatitis in pregnancy. *J. Pakistani Med. Assoc.*, **29**, 31–5
5. Khurol, M.S., Teli, M.R., Skidmore, S., Sofi, M.A. and Khuroo, M.I. (1981). *Am. J. Med.*, **70**, 252–5
6. Rizetto, M., Canese, M.G., Arico, S., Crivelli, O., Bonino, F., Trepo, C.G. and Verma, G. (1977). Immunofluorescence detection of a new antigen-antibody system (delta/anti-delta) associated to hepatitis B virus in liver and in serum of HBsAg carriers. *Gut*, **18**, 997–1003
7. Smedile, A., Dentico, P., Zanetti, A., Sagnelli, E., Nordenfelt, E., Actis, G.C. and Rizetto, M. (1981). Infection with the delta (?) agent in chronic HBsAg carriers. *Gastroenterology*, **81**, 992–7

8. Farci, P., Smedile, A., Lavarini, C., Piantino, P., Crivelli, O., Caporaso, N., Toti, M., Bonino, F. and Rizetto, M. (1983). Delta hepatitis in inapparent carriers of hepatitis B surface antigen. *Gastroenterology*, **85**, 669 – 73
9. Tong, M.J., Thursby, M., Rakela, J., McPeak, C., Edwards, V.M. and Mosley, J.W. (1981). *Gastroenterology*, **80**, 999 – 1004
10. Hoofnagle, J.H. and Alter, H.J. (1984). Chronic viral hepatitis. In Vyas, G.N., Dienstag, J.L. and Hoofnagle, J.H. (eds.) *Viral Hepatitis and Liver Disease*, pp. 97 – 111. (Orlando: Grune & Stratton, Inc.)
11. Shiraki, K., Yoshihara, N., Kawana, T., Yasui, J. and Sakurai, M. (1977). Hepatitis B surface antigen and chronic hepatitis in infants born to asymptomatic carrier mothers. *Am. J. Dis. Child.*, **131**, 644 – 7
12. Lee, A.K.Y., Ip, H.M.H. and Wong, V.C.W. (1978). Mechanisms of maternal – fetal transmission of hepatitis B virus. *J. Infect. Dis.*, **138**, 668 – 71
13. Derso, A., Boxall, E.H., Tarlow, M.J. and Flewett, T.H. (1978). Transmission of HBsAg from mother to infant in four ethnic groups. *Br. Med. J.*, **1**, 949-52
14. Stevens, C.E., Beasley, R.P., Tsui, J. and Lee, W.C. (1975). Vertical transmission of hepatitis B antigen in Taiwan. *N. Engl. J. Med.*, **292**, 771 – 4
15. Okada, K., Kamiyama, I., Inomata, M., Imai, M., Miyakawa, Y. and Maymi, M. (1976). e Antigen and anti-e in the serum of asymptomatic carrier mothers as indicators of positive and negative transmission of hepatitis B virus to their infants. *N. Engl. J. Med.*, **294**, 746 – 9
16. Stevens, C.E., Neurath, R.A., Beasley, R.P. and Szmuness, W. (1979). HBeAg and anti-HBe detection by radioimmunoassay: correlation with vertical transmission on hepatitis B virus in Taiwan. *J. Med. Virol.*, **3**, 237 – 41
17. Beasley, R.P., Hwang, L-Y, Lee, G.C.-Y., Lan, C., Huang, F. and Chen, C. (1983). Prevention of perinatally transmitted hepatitis B virus infections with hepatitis B immune globulin and hepatitis B vaccine. *Lancet*, **2**, 1099 – 102
18. Hollinger, F.B., Mosley, J.W., Szmuness, W., Aach, R.D., Peters, R.L. and Stevens, C. (1980). Transfusion-transmitted viruses study: experimental evidence for two non-A, non-B hepatitis agents. *J. Infect. Dis.*, **142**, 400 – 7
19. Dienstag, J.L. (1983). Non-A, non-B hepatitis. I. Recognition, epidemiology, and clinical features. *Gastroenterology*, **85**, 439 – 62
20. Knodell, R.G., Contad, M.E., Dienstag, J.L. and Bell, C.J. (1975). Etiological spectrum of post-transfusion hepatitis. *Gastroenterology*, **69**, 1278 – 85
21. Wick, M.R., Moore, S. and Taswell, H.F. (1985). Non-A, non-B hepatitis associated with blood transfusion. *Transfusion*, **25**, 93 – 101
22. Wong, D.C., Purcell, R.H., Sreenivasan, M.A., Prasad, S.R. and Pavri, K.M. (1980). Epidemic and endemic hepatitis in India: evidence for a non-A, non-B hepatitis virus aetiology. *Lancet*, **2**, 876 – 9
23. Enterically transmitted non-A, non-B hepatitis – East Africa. (1987). *Mortal. Morbid. Weekly*, **36**, 241 – 4
24. Enterically transmitted non-A, non-B hepatitis – Mexico. (1987). *Mortal. Morbid. Weekly*, **36**, 597 – 602
25. Kortez, R.L., Stone, O., Mousa, M. and Gitnick, G. (1985). Non-A, non-B post-transfusion hepatitis – a decade later. *Gastroenterology*, **88**, 1251 – 4
26. Gupta, B., Agarwal, S. and Joshi, V.V. (1978). Maternal/fetal transmission of HBsAg negative hepatitis (letter). *Lancet*, **2**, 740
27. Robinson, W.S. (1985). Hepatitis B virus. In Hollinger, F.B., Melnick, J.L. and Robinson, W.S. (eds.) *Viral Hepatitis*, pp. 19 – 56. (New York: Raven Press)
28. Werner, B.G., Dienstag, J.L., Kuter, B.J., Snydman, D.R., Polk, B.F., Craven, D.E., Platt, R., Crumpacker, C.S. and Grady, G.F. (1984). Immunologic responses to hepatitis B virus and their interpretations. In Millman, I., Eisenstein, R.K. and Blumberg, B.S. (eds.) *Hepatitis B: the Virus, the Disease, and the Vaccine*, pp. 105 – 11. (New York: Plenum Press)
29. Alter, H.J., Seeff, L.B., Kaplan, P.M., McAuliff, V.J., Wright, E.C., Gerlin, J.L., Purcell, R.H., Holland, P.V. and Zimmerman, H.J. (1976). Type B hepatitis: the infectivity of blood positive for e antigen and DNA polymerase after accidental needlestick exposure. *N. Engl. J. Med.*, **295**, 909 – 13

30. Beasley, R.P., Trepo, C., Stevens, C.E. and Szmuness, W. (1977). The e antigen and vertical transmission of hepatitis B surface antigen. *Am. J. Epidemiol.*, **105**, 94–8
31. Hieber, J.P., Dalton, D., Shorey, J. and Combes, B. (1977). Hepatitis and pregnancy. *J. Pediatr.*, **91**, 545–9
32. Shalev, E. and Bassan, H.M. (1982). Viral hepatitis during pregnancy in Israel. *Int. J. Gynecol. Obstet.*, **20**, 73–8
33. Schweitzer, I.L., Dunn, A.E.G., Peters, R.L. and Spears, R.L. (1973). Viral hepatitis B in neonates and infants. *Am. J. Med.*, **55**, 762–71
34. Gerety, R.J. and Schweitzer, I.L. (1977). Viral hepatitis type B during pregnancy, the neonatal period and infancy. *J. Pediatr.*, **90**, 368–74
35. Delaplane, D., Yogev, R., Crussi, F. and Shulman, S.T. (1983). Fatal hepatitis B in early infancy: the importance of identifying HBsAg-positive pregnant women and providing immunoprophylaxis to their newborns. *Pediatrics*, **72**, 176–80
36. Sinatra, F.R., Shah, P., Weissman, J.Y., Thomas, D.W., Merritt, R.J. and Tong, M.J. (1982). Perinatal transmitted acute icteric hepatitis B in infants born to hepatitis B surface antigen-positive and anti-hepatitis B e-positive carrier mothers. *Pediatrics*, **70**, 557–9
37. Wong, V.C.W., Lee, A.K.Y. and Ip, H.M.H. (1980). Transmission of hepatitis B antigens from symptom free carrier mothers to the fetus and the infant. *Br. J. Obstet. Gynaecol.*, **87**, 958–65
38. Maupas, P., Barin, F., Chiron, J.P., Coursaget, P., Goudeau, A., Perrin, J., Denise, F. and DiopMar, I. (1981). Efficacy of hepatitis B vaccine in prevention of early HBsAg carrier state in children. *Lancet*, **1**, 289–92
39. Beasley, R.P., Hwang, L-Y., Lin, C-C., Stevens, C.E., Wang, K-Y., Sun, T-S., Hsieh, F-J. and Szmuness, W. (1981). Hepatitis B immune globulin (HBIG) efficacy in the interruption of perinatal transmission of hepatitis B virus carrier state: initial report of a randomized double-blind placebo-controlled trial. *Lancet*, **2**, 388–93
40. Ohto, J., Lin, H-H., Kawana, T., Etoh, T. and Tohyama, H. (1987). Intrauterine transmission of hepatitis B virus is closely related to placental leakage. *J. Med. Virol.*, **21**, 1–6
41. Scott, R.M., Snitbhan, R., Bancroft, W.H., Alter, H.J. and Tingpalapong, M. (1980). Experimental transmission of hepatitis B virus by semen and saliva. *J. Infect. Dis.*, **142**, 67–71
42. Beasley, R.P. and Stevens, C.E. (1978). Vertical transmission of HBV and interruption with globulin. In Vyas, G.N., Cohen, S.N. and Schmid, R. (eds.) *Viral Hepatitis. Etiology Epidemiology, Pathogenesis and Prevention*, pp. 333–45. (Philadelphia: Franklin Institute Press)
43. Stokes, J. Jr., Berk, J.E., Malamut, L.L., Drake, M.E., Barondess, J.A., Bashe, W.J., Wolman, I.J., Farquhar, J.D., Bevan, B., Drummond, R.J., Maycock, Wd'A., Capps, R.B. and Bennett, A.M. (1954). The carrier state in viral hepatitis. *J. Am. Med. Assoc.*, **154**, 1059–65
44. Zanetti, A.R., Ferroni, P., Magliano, E.M., Pirovano, P., Lavarini, C., Massaro, A.L., Gavinelli, R., Fabris, C. and Rizzetto, M. (1982). Perinatal transmission of the hepatitis B virus and of the HBV-associated delta agent from mothers to offspring in Northern Italy. *J. Med. Virol.*, **9**, 139–48
45. Wong, V.C.W., Reesink, H.W., Ip, H.M.H., Lelie, P.N., Reerink-Brongers, E.E., Yeung, C.Y. and Ma, H.K. (1984). Prevention of the HBsAg carrier state in newborn infants of mothers who are chronic carriers of HBsAg and HBeAg by administration of hepatitis-B vaccine and hepatitis-B immunoglobulin. *Lancet*, **1**, 921–6
46. Tada, J., Yanagida, M., Mishina, J., Fujii, T., Baba, K., Ishikawa, S., Aihara, S., Tsuda, F., Miyakawa, Y. and Mayumi, M. (1982). Combined passive and active immunization of preventing perinatal transmission of hepatitis B virus carrier state. *Pediatrics*, **70**, 613–9
47. Stevens, C.E., Toy, P.T., Tong, M.J., Taylor, P.E., Vyas, G.N., Nair, P.V., Gusvalli, M. and Krugman, S. (1985). Perinatal hepatitis B virus transmission in the United States. Prevention by passive-active immunization. *J. Am. Med. Assoc.*, **253**, 1940–5
48. Reesink, H.W., Reerink-Brongers, E.E., Lafeber-Schut, B.J.T., Kalshoven-Benschop, J. and Brummelhuis, H.G.J. (1979). Prevention of chronic HBsAg carrier state in infants of

HBsAg-positive mothers by hepatitis B immunoglobulin. *Lancet*, **2**, 436 – 8
49. Inactivated hepatitis B virus vaccine. (1982). *Mortal. Morbid. Weekly*, **31**, 317 – 28
50. Recommendations for protection against viral hepatitis. (1985). *Mortal. Morbid. Weekly*, **34**, 313 – 35
51. Arevalo, J.A. and Washington, A.E. (1988). Cost-effectiveness of prenatal screening and immunization for hepatitis B virus. *J. Am. Med. Assoc.*, **259**, 365 – 9
52. 1986 Red Book. (1986). *Report of the Committee on Infectious Diseases*, pp. 178 – 91. (Elk Grove Village: American Academy of Pediatrics)
53. Barin, F., Denis, F., Chiron, J.P., Goudeau, A., Yvonnet, B., Coursaget, P. and DiopMar, I. (1982). Immune response in neonates to hepatitis B vaccine. *Lancet*, **1**, 251 – 3
54. Lee, G.C.-Y., Hwang, L-Y., Beasleym, R.P., Chen, S-H. and Lee, T-Y. (1983). Immunogenicity of hepatitis B virus vaccine in healthy Chinese neonates. *J. Infec. Dis.*, **148**, 526 – 9
55. Dienstag, J.L., Stevens, C.E., Bhan, J.A.K. and Szmuness, W. (1982). Hepatitis B vaccine administered to chronic carriers of hepatitis B surface antigen. *Ann. Intern. Med.*, **96**, 575 – 9
56. Lee, C., Han, D.G., Kim, P.K. and Chin, D.S. (1987). Transplacental transmission of hepatitis B (HB) virus: efficacy of vaccine for HBsAg positive infants at birth. *Pediatr. Res.*, **21**, 417A
57. Beasley, R.P., Stevens, C.E., Shiao, I-S. and Meng, H-C. (1975). Evidence against breastfeeding as a mechanism for vertical transmission of hepatitis B. *Lancet*, **2**, 740 – 1
58. Krugman, S. (1985). Viral hepatitis: 1985 update. *Pediatr. Rev.*, **7**, 3 – 11

14

AIDS in Pregnancy and the Newborn

Ellen Gould Chadwick

Although women account for only 7% of the total population of patients with the acquired immune deficiency syndrome (AIDS) in the United States, the vast majority of children with AIDS are the offspring of women with human immunodeficiency virus (HIV) infection. Fifty one percent of these women are black, 28% are white and 20% are Hispanic[1]. This racial distribution does not differ significantly from that of males infected through hetersexual activity or intravenous drug abuse (IVDA). By risk category, the largest proportion of women with AIDS are intravenous drug abusers (52%) followed by those with heterosexual contact with a person at risk for AIDS (21%), recipients of contaminated transfusions (10%), women born in a country where heterosexual transmission is common (6%), and women in whom epidemiologic data are incomplete or with no identified risk (11%)[1]. It has been estimated that approximately 75,000 intravenous drug-abusing women in the US are currently infected with HIV[2].

Because HIV infection appears to have little or no effect on fertility[3], the population of HIV-infected pregnant women will very likely continue to grow. Counseling and screening for HIV antibody should be offered to women of child-bearing age who are at risk for acquiring HIV infection (Table 14.1)[4]. Women who have a positive HIV antibody test should be counseled regarding their own risk of developing AIDS, and their capability to transmit the virus, both through sexual activity and to their offspring[4]. Their sexual partners should be encouraged to be tested, and, if negative, safe sex guidelines should be reviewed. Infected women should be advised to refrain from sharing needles/syringes or donating blood or organs, and they should notify anyone who may be in contact with their blood or body fluids, such as medical or dental professionals, of their HIV status. Although early case reports suggested that pregnancy may accelerate the development of clinical HIV disease[5], more recent comparative studies have shown no more rapid progression of disease during or shortly after gestation[6,7]. However, until more is known about the risk of perinatal HIV transmission, infected women should be encouraged to delay pregnancy.

191

There are three postulated routes by which perinatal HIV transmission occurs: (a) transplacental infection *in utero*, (b) exposure to blood and cervical secretions during delivery, and (c) postpartum ingestion of breast milk containing the virus. *In utero* HIV infection has been demonstrated by isolating the virus from aborted 15-and 20-week fetuses[8,9]. Perinatal infection has been suggested by Ho Pyun *et al.* who documented early neonatal synthesis of IgM and IgG_3 anti-HIV antibody following vaginal delivery by an infected mother[10]. The ability to recover HIV from cervical secretions further supports this route of transmission[11]. One infant reported by Ziegler *et al.* was presumed to have acquired HIV infection postnatally via breast milk, as the mother's only risk factor was a postpartum transfusion of blood from a donor subsequently found to have AIDS[12]. This potential mode of transmission clearly requires further investigation because it may have widespread and potentially devastating implications for developing countries in which breastfeeding is the cornerstone of infant nutrition and prophylaxis against diarrheal disease.

Table 14.1 Women who should be screened for HIV infection

---

1. Clinical evidence of HIV infection
2. Intravenous drug abusers
3. Women from countries where heterosexual transmission is common (Haiti, Central Africa)
4. Women with multiple sexual partners
5. Sexual partners of:
    a. bisexual men
    b. men with hemophilia
    c. men with evidence of HIV
    d. men from countries where heterosexual transmission is common

---

Adapted from reference 4

The rate of HIV transmission from infected mother to infant appears to be approximately $40-50\%$[13-15]. Among women who have already given birth to one child with HIV infection, $36-65\%$ of subsequent pregnancies have resulted in another infected infant[7,16,17]. However, determinants of maternal–fetal transmission are poorly defined. Clinical evidence of disease in the mother is not an important factor affecting transmission, as the majority of women giving birth to infants who are ultimately proved to have HIV infection are apparently healthy, although HIV antibody positive[16]. Viremia during gestation is an attractive hypothesized mode of transmitting the infection. However, Rogers *et al.* reported an infant who escaped infection despite isolation of HIV from the mother's peripheral lymphocytes throughout pregnancy and from the placenta at delivery[18]. The route of delivery does not appear to be crucial for infectivity as both caesarian and vaginal deliveries have produced HIV-infected infants[19,20]. Further complicating this picture are data regarding transmission of HIV in twin pairs. In two sets of dizygotic twins, infection occurred in all four offspring; however, in two sets of monozygotic twins, only one member of each twin pair was HIV-infected[17,21].

Current methods of HIV antibody detection do not allow definitive diagnosis of HIV infection in asymptomatic young infants. Virtually all neonates born to seropositive women are HIV antibody positive as a result of placental transfer of maternal IgG antibody[22]. Furthermore, such transplacentally-derived antibody may persist for up to 15 months of age[23]; this makes it difficult to demonstrate whether the infant is actively synthesizing anti-HIV in response to infection or merely has passively transmitted maternal antibody. Neonatal anti-HIV IgM may be absent[24] or only transiently present and, if present, may be directed against only a limited spectrum of epitopes[10]. Some infants may lose maternal antibody and not develop endogenous antibody for as long as twelve months[25]. Other infants have become seronegative within the first few months of life, and never develop detectable levels of HIV antibody, despite having a positive viral culture or repeated HIV antigenemia[20,26-28].

Clearly, conventional serologic tests for HIV antibody are of very limited value in accurate detection of HIV-infected infants less than 15 months of age. Although viral culture or HIV antigen detection should be preferable methods to identify infected infants, the sensitivity of these procedures must be improved. The ability to recover virus is limited by transcriptional viral dormancy and the small number of infected cells. For example, in a series of 9 children known to be infected by previous culture or antigen tests, only 7 of 19 repeat viral cultures were positive[20]. Furthermore, because of the specific protective requirements for handling HIV isolates, few laboratories are equipped to provide viral culture techniques for routine clinical diagnostic purposes. Although HIV antigenemia has been demonstrated in young infants[29], it is generally not detectable in neonates, presumably because it is bound by the high levels of circulating maternal antibody[30].

Although the vast majority of infants who ultimately prove to be HIV-infected are asymptomatic at birth[30], there is controversy over this issue. Marion et al. recently reported a dysmorphic syndrome hypothesized to be related to intrauterine HIV infection in 20 randomly selected children with AIDS[31]. The features of the syndrome include growth failure, microcephaly, ocular hypertelorism, prominent box-like forehead, mild obliquity of the eyes, long palpebral fissure with blue sclera, short nose with flattened columella and well-formed triangular philtrum and patulous lips.

However, these features were not compared with a control population of infants born to drug-abusing mothers without HIV infection. Furthermore, two studies from New York and Africa that evaluated a total of 57 HIV-positive children and 49 controls found no dysmorphism which identified perinatal HIV exposure[32,33].

Laboratory evidence of immune dysfunction during the newborn period is also generally lacking. Specifically, the hallmarks of HIV infection, such as hypergammaglobulinemia, diminished CD4 positive cells, reversed T-lymphocyte subset ratio, and anemia, are strikingly absent in infected neonates[30]. The above abnormalities become more pronounced as HIV infection progresses. The majority of infants with HIV infection become symptomatic within the first two years of life, with the mean onset of symptoms at approximately 6 months of age[30,34]. Infants may present with a variety of non-specific symptoms such as failure to thrive, chronic diarrhea, oral thrush, hepatosplenomegaly or lymphadenopathy; or they may develop an opportunistic infection such as *P. carinii* pneumonia, disseminated candidiasis, cytomegalovirus, or herpes simplex or zoster infections. Recurrent bacterial infections, lymphoid interstitial pneumonitis and chronic encephalopathy are common in HIV infection in children. The reader is referred to several excellent review articles for an overview of the clinical findings in symptomatic pediatric HIV disease[17,23,35]. In summary, the diversity of symptomatology in pediatric HIV infection makes it important to have a high index of suspicion for the disease. A thorough history from the mother should help to elucidate possible risk factors which would predispose her, and subsequently her infant, to HIV infection. Appropriate counseling regarding reduction of risk behaviors and perinatal transmission issues is at present our best weapon against a growing population of children with AIDS.

REFERENCES

1. Guinan, M.E. and Hardy, A. (1987). Epidemiology of AIDS in women in the United States. *J. Am. Med. Assoc.*, **257**, 2039–42
2. Wofsy, C.B. (1987). *Report Of The Surgeon General's Workshop on Children with HIV Infection and Their Families*, April 6–9, pp. 32–34
3. Selwyn, P.A., Feingold, A.R., Schoenbaum, E.E., Davenny, K., Robertson, V. and Shulman, J. (1987). Pregnancy outcome and HIV infection in intravenous drug abusers. Presented at the *III International Conference on AIDS*, June 1–5, 1987, Washington DC
4. Centers for Disease Control. (1986). Recommendations for assisting in the prevention of perinatal transmission of HTLV-III/LAV and acquired immunodeficiency syndrome. *J. Am. Med. Assoc.*, **255**, 25–31
5. Minkoff, H., Nanda, D., Menez, R. and Fikrig, S. (1987). Pregnancies resulting in infants with acquired immunodeficiency syndrome or AIDS-related complex: follow-up of mothers, children and subsequently born siblings. *Obstet. Gynecol.*, **69**, 288–91

194

6. Ciraru-Vigneron, N., Tan Lung, R.N., Brunner, C., Barrier, J., Wautier, J.L. and Boizard, B. (1987). HIV infection among high-risk pregnant women. *Lancet*, **2**, 630
7. Nachman, S. (1987). Human immunodeficiency virus (HIV) infection during pregnancy: a longitudinal study. Presented at the *III International Conference on AIDS*. June 1-5, 1987, Washington DC
8. Sprecher, S., Soumernkoff, Puissant, F. and Dugueldre, M. (1986). Vertical transmission of HIV in 15 week fetus. *Lancet*, **2**, 288-89
9. Jovaisas, E., Koch, M.A., Schafer, A., Stauber, M. and Lowenthal, D. (1985). LAV/HTVL III in 20-week fetus. *Lancet*, **2**, 1129
10. Ho Pyun, K., Ochs, H.D., Dufford, M.T.W. and Wedgwood, R.J. (1987). Perinatal infection with human immunodeficiency virus: specific antibody responses by the neonate. *N. Engl. J. Med.*, **317**, 611-14
11. Vogt, M.W., Witt, D.J., Craven, D.E., Byington, R., Crawford, D.F., Schooley, R.T. and Hirsch, M.S. (1986). Isolation of HTLV-III/LAV from cervical secretions of women at risk for AIDS. *Lancet*, **1**, 525-27
12. Ziegler, J.B., Johnson, R.O., Cooper, D.A. and Gold, J. (1985). Postnatal transmission of AIDS-associated retrovirus from mother to infant. *Lancet*, **2**, 896-97
13. De Maria, A., Varnier, O.E. and Melica, G. (1987). Transmission of HTLV III (HIV) in infants of seropositive mothers. Presented at the *III International Conference on AIDS*, June 1-5, 1987, Washington DC
14. Johnson, J.P., Alger, L., Nair, P., Watkins, S., Jett, K. and Alexander, S. (1987). HIV screening in the high risk obstetric population and infant serologic analysis. Presented at the *III International Conference on AIDS*, June 1-5, 1987, Washington DC
15. Semprini, E., Vucetich, A. and Pardi, G. (1987). HIV infection and AIDS in newborn babies of mothers positive for HTV antibody. *Br. Med. J.*, **294**, 610
16. Scott, G.B., Mastrucci, M.T., Hutto, S.C. and Parks, W.P. (1987). Mothers of infants with HIV infection: outcome of subsequent pregnancies. Presented at the *III International Conference on AIDS*. June 1-5. 1987, Washington DC
17. Rubinstein, A. (1986). Pediatric aids. *Curr. Probl. Pediatr.*, **16**, 361-409
18. Rogers, M.F., Ewing, E.P. Jr. and Warfield, D. (1986). Virologic studies of HTLV-III/LAV in pregnancy: case report of a woman with AIDS. *Obstet. Gynecol.*, **685**, 25-65
19. Thomas, P.A., O'Donnell, R.E. and Guigli, P. (1987). Gestational characteristics and mode of delivery of 98 children with AIDS in New York City. Presented at the *III International Conference on AIDS*. June 1-5, 1987, Washington DC
20. Mok, J.Q., De Rossi, A., Ades, A.E., Giaquinto, C., Grosch-Worner, I. and Peckham, C.S. (1987). Infants born to mothers seropositive for human immunodeficiency virus. *Lancet*, **2**, 1164-68
21. Menez-Bautista, R., Fikrig, S.M., Pahwa, S., Sarangadharan, M.G. and Stoneburner, R.L. (1986). Monozygotic twins discordant for the acquired immunodeficiency syndrome. *Am. J. Dis. Child.*, **140**, 678-79
22. Kreiss, J.K., Quinn, T., Nidinya-Achola, J., Vercauteren, G. and Plummer, F.A. (1987). Congenital transmission of HIV in Nairobi, Kenya. Presented at the *III International Conference on AIDS*, June 1-5, 1987, Washington DC
23. Centers for Disease Control (1987). Classification system for human immunodeficiency virus (HIV) infection in children under 13 years of age. *Mortal. Morbid. Weekly Rev.*, **36**, 225-35
24. Johnson, J.P., Nair, P. and Alexander, S. (1987). Early diagnosis of HIV infection in the neonate. *N. Engl. J. Med.*, **316**, 273-74
25. Aiuti, F., Luzi, G., Mezzaroma, I., Scano, G. and Papetti, C. (1987). Delayed appearance of HIV infection in children. *Lancet*, **2**, 658
26. Borkowsky, W., Paul, D., Bebenroth, D., Krasinski, K., Moore, T. and Chandwani, S. (1987). Human-immunodeficiency-virus infections in infants negative for anti-HIV by enzyme-linked immunoassay. *Lancet*, **2**, 1168-71
27. Lange, J.M.A., Paul, D.A. and Huisman, H.G. (1986). Persistent HIV antigenaemia and decline of HIV core antibodies associated with transmission to AIDS. *Br. Med. J.*, **293**, 1459-62

28. Grosch-Worner, I., Koch, S., Stuck, B., Vocks, M. and Woweries, J. (1987). Study of children born to HIV (human immunodeficiency virus) positive mothers. Presented at the *European Society for Pediatric Research*, Sept. 6–10, Padova, Italy

29. Borkowsky, W., Krasinski, K.K., Paul, D., Lawrence, R., Moore, T. and Candwanl, S. (1987). Retroviral antigenemia in children with HIV infection. Presented at the *III International Conference on AIDS*, June 1–5, 1987, Washington DC

30. Blanche, S., Rouzioux, C., Veber, F., DeDeist, F., Mayaux, M.J. and Griscelli, C. (1987). Prospective study on newborn of HIV seropositive women. Presented at the *III International Conference on AIDS*, June 1–5, 1987, Washington DC

31. Marion, R.W., Winania, A.A., Hutcheon, G. and Rubinstein, A. (1986). Human T-cell lymphotrophic virus type III (HTLV III) embryopathy. *Am. J. Dis. Child.*, **140**, 638–40

32. Embree, J., Braddick, M., Ndiyna-Achola, J., Low, B., Murithii, J. and Hoff, C. (1987). Does prenatal human immunodeficiency virus (HIV) infection produce infant malformations? Presented at the *III International Conference on AIDS*, June 1–5, 1987, Washington DC

33. Qazi, Q.H., Sheikh, T.M., Fikrig, S. and Menikoff, H. (1987). Lack of evidence for craniofacial dysmorphism in perinatal human immunodeficiency virus infection. *J. Pediatr.*, **112**, 7–11

34. Rogers, M.F., Thomas, P.A., Starcher, E.T., Noa, M.C., Bush, T.J. and Jaffe, H.W. (1987). Acquired immunodeficiency syndrome in children: report on the Centers for Disease Control national surveillance, 1982 to 1985. *Pediatrics*, **79**, 1008–14

35. Pahwa, S., Kaplan, M., Fikrig, S., Pahwa, R., Sarngadharan, M.G., Popovic, M. and Gallo, R.C. (1986). Spectrum of human T-cell lymphotropic virus type III infection in children. *J. Am. Med. Assoc.*, **255**, 2299–3005

Appendix

Suggested Protocol for Reporting and Management of Suspect Drug/Alcohol-Related Child Abuse and Neglect*

I.   PRENATAL PERIOD

A. When a patient presents to the prenatal clinics with an acknowledged history of drug/alcohol abuse, without signs and/or symptoms:
   (1) If the patient appears to be psychosocially low risk, (see Section IV) no action needs to be taken other than charting a history of drug/alcohol abuse in the patient's medical record.
   (2) If the patient appears to be psychosocially high risk (see Section IV.A):
      (a) A toxic screen shall be ordered at the discretion of the physician only with the verbal consent of the patient.
      (b) The patient's verbal consent to a toxic screen procedure must be documented in the patient's medical records.
      (c) If the patient declines the toxic screen, this should also be noted in the patient's medical records.
      (d) Refer the patient to clinical social work.

B. When a pregnant woman presents to the prenatal clinic with signs and/or symptoms of drug/alcohol abuse:
   (1) Refer the patient to clinical social work.
   (2) The physician shall order a toxic screen, if medically indicated, regardless of the patient's consent. Following the toxic screen results:

---

* Adapted from UCLA Medical Center and Northwestern Memorial Hospital policy for management of potential drug/alcohol-related child abuse/neglect in the perinatal period.

(a) If the screen is positive for:
  (i) Alcohol – follow-up by social worker or public health nurse.
  (ii) Controlled or illegal substances and/or chemicals (including, but not limited to, PCP, methadone, barbituates, heroin, cocaine):
    – Prescribed appropriate use – no further action needs to be taken.
    – Prescribed and inappropriate use – follow-up by social worker or public health nurse.
    – Unprescribed use – follow-up by child abuse or chemical dependence team.
(b) If the screen is negative, or the patient declines a toxic screen, refer the patient to social worker or public health nurse.
(3) A repeat screen must be obtained at the time of delivery.

C. When the father of the unborn child, or the significant other of the pregnant patient, is suspected of drug/alcohol abuse, refer the case to social worker or public health nurse for initiation of referral for treatment and counseling. Home visit as needed to follow-up and assess the home situation.

D. Despite positive drug/alcohol screens, only extreme and dangerous situations are reported to child protection services during the prenatal period. Efforts are directed at counseling the parent(s) and making appropriate referrals for treatment.

II. LABOR AND DELIVERY

A. When a patient presents to the Delivery Room with an acknowledged history of drug/alcohol abuse, without signs and/or symptoms:
  (1) If the patient appears to be psychosocially low risk (see Section IV.B) the physician in collaboration with the Delivery Room nurses, shall:
    (a) Consider a toxic screen at the physician's discretion, if medically indicated.
    (b) Refer the patient to social work.
  (2) If the patient appears to be psychosocially high risk (see Section IV.B):
    (a) A toxic screen shall be ordered (follow the same procedures as for IV.B.2).
    (b) Refer the patient to social worker.

B. When a pregnant woman presents to the Delivery Room with signs and/or symptoms of drug/alcohol abuse, with or without an acknowledged history of such abuse:
   (1) The physician shall order a toxic screen.
   (2) The physician, in collaboration with the Delivery Room nurses, shall refer the patient to social work and the child-abuse team.

III. POSTNATAL PERIOD

A. A pediatrician shall order a toxic screen on any neonate:
   (1) Born to a mother with an acknowledged history of drug/alcohol abuse.
   (2) Born to a mother with signs and/or symptoms suggestive of drug/alcohol abuse.
   (3) Born with signs and/or symptoms suggestive of maternal drug/alcohol abuse.

B. After the toxic screen results are obtained, the following action shall be taken:
   (1) If the toxic screen for the neonate is positive for:
      (a) Alcohol
         (i) Refer the case to social work.
         (ii) Refer to the child abuse team and report to the state child protection services.
      (b) Controlled or illegal substances and/or chemicals (including, but not limited to PCP, heroin, cocaine):
         (i) Prescribed and appropriate use – no further action needs to be taken.
         (ii) Prescribed and inappropriate use – refer the case to social work and the child-abuse team.
         (iii) Unprescribed use – refer to child-abuse team and report to State child protection services.
   (2) If the toxic screen for the neonate is negative, but drug withdrawal is suspected, or if the infant is symptomatic, physician or neonatal nurse shall refer the case to social work, the child-abuse team and child protection services.
   (3) If the toxic screen for the neonate is negative and the infant is not symptomatic:
      (a) The physician or neonatal nurse shall refer the case to social work.
      (b) The health care team shall provide discharge planning to insure follow-up care for the infant.

IV. PSYCHOSOCIAL HIGH RISK

A. Prenatal indicators:
  (1) The mother conceals or denies the pregnancy.
  (2) Abortion is unsuccessfully sought or attempted.
  (3) Relinquishment for adoption is sought, then reversed.
  (4) History of severe marital discord.
  (5) No preparation for receiving the baby.
  (6) Parent(s) without support system.
  (7) History of serious mental illness, institutionalization, current depression, or repeated foster homes in either parent.
  (8) History of violent behavior or serious prison or jail or juvenile detention sentence in either parent.
  (9) History of previous abuse or neglect of another child.
  (10) Consistently avoids or misses medical appointments and is noncompliant.

B. Delivery Room indicators:
  (1) Review above Prenatal Indicators.
  (2) Hostile reaction or avoidance of contact, verbal or non-verbal – inappropriate verbalizations, glances, no eye contact, disparaging remarks, pulling away.
  (3) Disappointment over sex and appearance of the baby.
  (4) Negative interaction between baby, mother and significant other.

C. Postnatal Indicators
  (1) Review above Prenatal and Delivery Room Indicators.
  (2) Lack of behaviors indicating maternal attachment and bonding:
      (a) Doesn't want to hold, feed or name the baby.
      (b) Avoids eye contact and touch.
      (c) No signs of cuddling or talking to the baby.
      (d) Disparaging remarks about the baby.
      (e) The mother feeds her baby in a mechanical or other inappropriate way.
      (f) Spanking of the newborn or overt anger directed toward him/her.
  (2) The mother attempts to sign her sick newborn out of the hospital against medical advice.
  (3) A postpartum depression.
  (4) Suspicious early departure of mother from hospital.
  (5) Inadequate visiting or telephone patterns if mother is discharged before the baby.
  (6) Reluctance to come in for the baby when his/her discharge is approved.

Index